READINGS FOR A NEW PUBLIC HEALTH

Edited by
CLAUDIA J. MARTIN
and
DAVID V. McQUEEN

READINGS FOR
A NEW PUBLIC HEALTH

EDINBURGH UNIVERSITY PRESS

© Edinburgh University Press 1989
22 George Square, Edinburgh

Set in Linoterm Times Roman
by Speedspools, Edinburgh, and
printed in Great Britain by
J. W. Arrowsmith Limited,
Bristol

British Library Cataloguing
   in Publication Data
Readings for a new public health
1. Man. Health. Social aspects
I. Martin, Claudia J. II. McQueen, David V.
362.'042
ISBN 0 85224 598 x
ISBN 0 85224 616 1 pbk

CONTENTS

CONTRIBUTORS

AMANDA AMOS
Department of Community Medicine, University of Edinburgh
JOHN ASHTON
Department of Community Health, University of Liverpool
KATHRYN BACKETT
Research Unit in Health and Behavioural Change, University of Edinburgh
MEL BARTLEY
Department of Social Policy, University of Edinburgh
FRANK BECHHOFER
Research Centre for Social Sciences, University of Edinburgh
GRAHAM BICKLER
Department of Community Medicine, Camberwell Health Authority
DAVID BLANE
Behavioural Science Unit, Charing Cross and Westminster Medical School
DAVID CILL-MHUIRE
Community Health Resource Unit, Glasgow
SARAH CURTIS AND SOPHIE HYNDMAN
Department of Geography and Earth Science, Queen Mary College, London
NEIL DRUMMOND
West Granton Community Health Project, Edinburgh
PAMELA GILLIES
Department of Community Medicine and Epidemiology, University of Nottingham
PAULINE GINNETY, JANE WILDE AND MARY BLACK
Health Education Department, EHSSB, Belfast
GRAHAM HART
Department of Genito-Urinary Medicine, Middlesex Hospital Medical School
SONJA HUNT
Research Unit in Health and Behavioural Change, University of Edinburgh
ANTONIA INESON
Lothian Health Education Department, Edinburgh

ROSEMARIE KLESSE AND UTE SONNTAG
Bremen Institute for Prevention Research and Social Medicine, Bremen, FRG

RONALD LABONTE
Toronto Department of Public Health, Toronto, Canada

JULIAN LITTLE
Department of Community Medicine and Epidemiology, University of Nottingham

SALLY MACINTYRE AND STUDY TEAM
MRC Medical Sociology Unit, Glasgow

DAVID McQUEEN
Research Unit in Health and Behavioural Change, University of Edinburgh

CLAUDIA MARTIN
Research Unit in Health and Behavioural Change, University of Edinburgh

LESLEY MORRISON
Department of Community Medicine, City of London and Hackney Health Authority

MICHEL O'NEILL
Ecole des Sciences Infirmières, Université Laval, Quebec, Canada

BERNARD PISSARO
Faculté de Médecine, St Antoine, Paris

JENNIE POPAY
Thomas Coram Research Unit, Institute of Education, London

HEATHER ROBERTS
Department of Community Medicine and Epidemiology, University of Nottingham

ALEX SCOTT-SAMUEL
Department of Community Medicine, Liverpool Health Authority

JEAN SPRAY AND KAREN GREENWOOD
Health Education Department, Paddington and North Kensington Health Authority

ALF TROJAN
Institut für Medizinische Soziologie, University of Hamburg, FRG

CHRISTINA VICTOR
Department of Community Medicine, St Mary's Hospital, London

CHRISTEL ZENKER
Bremen Institute for Prevention Research and Social Medicine, Bremen, FRG

Introduction

1

CLAUDIA MARTIN AND DAVID MCQUEEN

FRAMEWORK FOR A NEW PUBLIC HEALTH

Introduction

The efforts to establish a 'new public health' should be seen in the context of the public health in general. In Anglo-Saxon cultures, public health has a rich and varied history although it is necessary to distinguish the public health movement from the development, establishment and growth of public health institutions.

Rosen (1958) has traced this history in some detail. Set in the broader context of the European work of Virchow and Grotjahn, British concern with public health centred around a response to the implications of large-scale industrial and economic changes taking place in Britain. For example, Kay's work (1832) emphasised the impact of industrial conditions on the public health. This and other writing laid the foundation for the work of Chadwick and other legendary heroes of nineteenth-century public health. Many historians would come to view this work as the foundation for present day social medicine in Britain. It is not the purpose of this chapter to detail the route from Chadwick to the chair of social medicine at Edinburgh, but merely to recognise this linkage and emphasise that it is part of the historical legend which colours the view of public health in Britain. In many ways the case could be made that any continuity of beliefs is mainly through the biomedical sciences with relatively little emphasis on the social sciences, either in the nineteenth or twentieth centuries.

Social medicine as a concept came much later, if at all, to the United States. None-the-less, it arose from many of the same concerns with housing, the effects of industrialisation, the need for better nutrition and for social welfare. The repository for the concerns of social medicine are largely found in the discipline of medical sociology in the US.

Whether one views the broad sweep of social medicine in Britain or medical sociology in the US, the legacy has been a concern with the social context of health, albeit from a largely biomedical perspective. Thus, the present-day institutions, whether departments of community medicine in Britain or schools of public health in the US, which have inherited the mantle of public health, are founded in social ideology, but are largely without a social science base. The dominant disciplines are those of epidemiology, biostatistics and pathobiology. The principle areas of study are chronic and infectious diseases and the analysis of medical care services. The social and behavioural sciences of anthropology, sociology, psychology and political science remain generally weak within such institutions. Of course, this is a gross generalisation. Readers may cite exceptions, but that is precisely the point.

The growing awareness of the discrepancy between the received ideology about what constitutes public health and the current practice and institutionalisation of public health has led to a movement to create a 'new public health' that is concerned with both the public and with health; this emphasis shifts the focus from patients and hospitals to people and their everyday life.

This movement was foreshadowed by many subtle changes which took place during the 1970s and early 1980s. Some changes are reflected in the heady debate over names of fields of study. Is it medical psychology or health psychology, medical sociology or the sociology of health, health education or health promotion? Even the biomedically based fields like epidemiology began to consider social factors as risk factors, culminating in concern with such clearly psychosocial constructs as social support, coping, isolation, etc. Studies of 'lifestyle' and 'health' began to flow from epidemiologists. Suddenly working conditions, eating habits and other behaviours were fashionable in the etiology of chronic diseases. Clearly, public health was changing.

The 'new public health' now appears as the next stage. It has a divided legacy: the public health ideology or mythology of the nineteenth century fused with the rapid changes of the past two decades. Much of this movement crystallised in the international meeting 'An International Conference on Health Promotion: The Move Towards a New Public Health' in Ottawa (1986). The very fact that such a large meeting could be sustained around such a theme made it clear that a 'new public health' was on the health agenda. This book of readings should be seen in light of this changing view of what constitutes the public health. The readings reflect not only the embryonic nature of this somewhat amorphous entity called the new public health, but also many issues and problems raised and unresolved. What are some of these issues and problems associated with a time of transition?

First, there is the problem of research one would like to do as opposed to the real world constraints on such research. These constraints come not only from institutions, but from within the research community itself. Thus, much research, including that illustrated in this book, starts with ideologies and premises which reflect the new public health but carries out research which is very much in the traditional mould of the old public health. Clearly there is a mismatch between ideology and technique. The technique is biomedically based. Inherently, most research designs, whether in the social or biomedical sciences, start with the researcher in control of how the research should be conducted. This is part of the power which a researcher is unlikely easily to yield. The uncomfortable fact remains that 'top-down' research sits comfortably in the research ethos. So, there is little tradition and knowledge of how a researcher could even begin to design and carry out a 'bottom-up' approach. Indeed, the fact that researchers even see themselves as the top looking down illustrates one of the dilemmas of the new public health. That is, how can community action be enabled without direction? The translation of research findings into policy formulation and action is a further crucial hurdle and will, perhaps, require greater motivation on the part of researchers to disseminate findings beyond obscure journals and supportive peer groups.

Current perspectives

Public health measures over the last century, such as improved sanitation, Clean Air and Housing Acts have all contributed to a markedly healthier population (McKeown and Lowe, 1966). Mass immunisation programmes have also helped diminish (or even eradicate) the impact of formerly fatal or crippling diseases. Whereas medicine is largely concerned with the diagnosis and treatment of individual illnesses (or, perhaps more accurately, the illnesses and diseases affecting individuals), public health is mainly concerned with prevention and diminution of illness and disease in the population. Early public health actions were mostly extrinsic to formal health care focusing instead on living conditions and environmental factors. In recent years, however, prevention has increasingly come to mean the prevention of illness in individuals by focusing on personal behaviour. The 'risk factor' approach, whereby individuals' presumed probability of developing a particular disease is characterised in terms of their profile with respect to specific behavioural or lifestyle factors, has become an accepted approach. This is demonstrated by several large-scale intervention programmes designed to reduce the prevalence of specific diseases through attempts to reduce the prevalence of particular behaviours in the population (for example, The Multiple Risk Factor Intervention Trial (MRFIT) in the USA, and The North Karelia Project in Finland – both concerned with reducing coronary heart disease (CHD)). There is, however, no unambiguous evidence that these trials have had any measurable success which could be directly attributed to their actions. Heart disease often did decline in project target areas over the course of trial periods, but frequently no more than in the countries as a whole. What did occur in each country was a general improvement in living and working conditions of the populations concerned.

Heart disease, like almost all disease categories, is strongly associated with social class. A study of CHD mortality rates among different civil service grades found that higher status or grade was linked with lower CHD mortality; the traditional risk factors for CHD (diet, smoking and exercise) only accounted for a small part of the variations in relative risk of CHD mortality (Rose and Marmot, 1981). However, the individualising of health and illness has, in effect, removed the social dimension from consideration of disease causation and, hence, from prevention (Bartley, 1985). It also implies that ill-health can be characterised in terms of single factor, disease-specific causality rather than in terms of a general model of susceptibility to ill-health. Yet, health experience – whether assessed in terms of morbidity or mortality – is strongly related to social factors. Although personal behaviours may contribute to ill-health, most activities are themselves socially structured and determined.

The persistence of socially structured inequalities in health, documented forcibly in the UK by *The Black Report* (Townsend and Davidson, 1982) and more recently by *The Health Divide* (Whitehead, 1987) have led to many questions about the effectiveness of biomedical models of prevention and health care. Despite overall improvements in standards of living, relative material disadvantage and great inequalities in employment, income and housing persist. The effects on health of unemployment, poor housing and low income are well documented (e.g.

Platt and Kreitman, 1985; Martin *et al.*, 1987; Fox and Shewry, 1988). Not only physical, but also mental health is influenced by social factors (Brown and Harris, 1978). Clearly, health cannot be promoted without reference to structural factors and health promotion activities must extend beyond formal health services.

A new public health movement, concerned with the effects of social conditions and relationships on physical and mental health has emerged in several countries over the last decade. This movement is re-focusing attention on those factors which are largely beyond individual control, and broadens health concerns beyond health care provision. This book of Readings looks at some of the main issues confronting a new public health. All of the papers included reflect some or all of these issues; the placing of each paper under a specific heading is mainly for convenience and merely indicates the dominant theme contained in the paper.

Agendas for a new public health. The new public health movement has theoretical, political, ideological and practical components. The first set of papers is intended to demonstrate some of the principal issues which require serious consideration in establishing a new public health. These include: the historical background of the public health movement and its relevance for current debates; inequalities in health and the social patterning of health and illness; the role of information in promoting healthy practices; co-operation between professional and administrative groups; the need for changes in professional rather than laye behaviour; the formulation and implementation of health-relevant programmes and policies; and the need to develop adequate and appropriate research techniques, both to assess needs and to evaluate health promotion programmes.

Inequalities in health. Although it is well-documented that social and economic disadvantage is linked to health experience, basic research is needed which examines links between specific factors and health outcome, and explores health inequalities among different groups in the population. The predictability with which socio-economic status is associated with almost *all* health outcomes needs to be underlined. Although social class based on the Registrar General's Classification of Occupations is a crude measure (Cameron and Jones, 1984), it nevertheless appears to reflect pervasive health differences within the population (MacIntyre, 1986).

The components of disadvantage reflected in the associations

between class and health are obviously crucial. While such fragmen-
tation has its attendant dangers – possibly diverting attention from
the complex and cumulative effects of deprivation and implying that
limited changes will suffice – arguments for structural, economic
and social change require detailed documentation. This is necessary
if only to counter arguments that such associations are artefactual,
the result of social selection factors, or merely a consequence of the
unhealthy individual actions of sub-sections of the population. The
Black Report considered each of these options and concluded that
health inequalities are largely materially based (Blane, 1985).

Personal behaviour and public health. There is little doubt that
certain behaviours can be health-damaging, increasing the risk of
pathology. Obvious examples are the association between cigarette
smoking and lung cancer, first demonstrated by Doll (e.g. Doll and
Hill, 1964), and associations between smoking in pregnancy and
low birth weight and perinatal mortality (Simpson, 1957). Yet even
here, the relationships between the behaviour and the outcomes are
complex and it is quite clear that social factors must play a part in the
aetiology of lung cancer (Sterling, 1978) and poor perinatal outcome (Rush and Cassano, 1983). Nevertheless, a highly individualised view of illness causation, with attendant overtones of 'victim-
blaming', has come to be an accepted model and underpins many
health education endeavours.

Much of epidemiological research has focused on, what might be
termed, 'the holy four' of personal behaviours – namely, smoking,
alcohol consumption, diet and exercise (McQueen, 1988). Rarely
is attention paid to the social context in which behaviours develop
and are maintained, or to other behaviours which may be important for health. Personal behaviours do not exist in isolation, but
are related in complex ways to the social and economic structure
and the constraints of daily life. The papers in this section reflect
the diversity of health behaviour research which incorporate these
social dimensions.

Information and the public health. There has long been a tradition
that the lay public should not have access to certain kinds of information about their own health. This is evidenced, for example, by
the 'confidentiality' of medical records which any medical practitioner (and for that matter, any medical receptionist) may see but
which the patient concerned cannot (Lovell, 1987). It is also apparent in the kinds of official health information which is disseminated
in, for instance, health education material and media campaigns.

What is lacking is easily available information about environmental hazards and their possible effect on health.

The amount, form, substance and dissemination of information relevant to health plays an important role in the new public health movement. It is predicated on the assumption that people have a right of access to information about a range of issues – be it the effects of radiation or hazards in the home and workplace. Implicit in a more open approach to health information, is the view that the lay public are not passive consumers or recipients of official edicts but can determine, for themselves, the risks they might face, and can be trusted to act responsibly with information concerning the health of their environment.

Professional behaviour: new roles and structures. Health care delivery is no longer confined to the doctor's surgery or to medical practitioners. Increasingly, health promotion activities take place in 'the community', the workplace and the home. A public health approach has necessitated a reappraisal of the role and remit of professional health workers and of the ways in which health promotion programmes can be developed and implemented. Consideration has to be given to lay views and local concerns, the political implications of health promotion work cannot be ignored, and service delivery must be restructured. The papers included in this section are concerned with some of these wider issues and how they impinge on those attempting to change the public health.

Community health initiatives. The Declaration of Alma Ata contained the statement that: 'The people have a right and duty to participate individually and collectively in the planning and implementation of their health care' (WHO, 1978). This view was further endorsed at a subsequent WHO conference organised around the theme of healthy public policy. The resulting Ottawa Charter For Health Promotion stated that: 'Health promotion works through concrete and effective community action. . . . At the heart of this process is the empowerment of communities . . . Community development draws on existing human and material resources in the community to enhance self-help and social support, and to develop flexible systems for strengthening public participation and direction of health matters.'

The development of programmes directed from the bottom (i.e. the community) rather than from the top (i.e. the professionals), in which the views of the public are not only represented but are paramount, is the subject of this final section. The papers included here all describe different attempts to implement the ideals of participation, co-operation, lay perception and social action. These initiatives are largely unconcerned with targeting specific individual behaviours; nor are they usually concerned with the prevention of specific diseases. Instead they involve health promotion in a wider sense: by involving the local population in decisions about the direction and form of any intervention; by providing resources such as health information, support for self-help groups and counselling; and providing a forum for debate about local health issues.

A healthy scepticism?

The principles expressed in the Ottawa Charter represent a possible ideal for health promotion; their achievement is inevitably more problematic. It could be argued, for example, that community-based initiatives have merely resulted in the replacement of one set of professionals (medical practitioners) with another (e.g. sociologist, community worker) and that the lay public is as excluded as ever. Issues of evaluation are rarely addressed. Are these efforts actually successful in involving the public? Do they promote health? Perhaps the essence of a new public health is a healthy scepticism about the role that health professionals, whether biomedically or behaviourally based, can play in the reduction and amelioration of ill-health which is to a large degree a consequence of a modern industrialised world and its social structure.

An international conference 'Changing the Public Health', organised by the Research Unit in Health and Behavioural Change of Edinburgh University and The Scottish Health Education Group, was held in Edinburgh in October 1987. The aim of the conference was to emphasise the importance of a public health perspective in the promotion of health. This book of Readings is based, in part, on papers presented at that meeting. The papers represent the ideas of many disciplines and the Readings reflect this diversity which is in the spirit of a new public health. It is not intended that that this book should simply be conference proceedings. Rather, the edited papers exemplify the main issues confronting a new public health movement and provide examples of the way forward in this important development in health promotion.

References

Bartley, M. (1985) Coronary heart disease and the public health 1850–1983, *Sociology of Health and Illness 7*, 289–313.

Blane, D. (1985) An assessment of the Black Report's explanation of health inequalities, *Sociology of Health and Illness 7*, 423–45.

Brown, G. W. and Harris, T. O. (1978) *Social Origins of Depression*, London: Tavistock Publications.

Cameron, D. and Jones, I. G. (1984) Social class analysis – an embarrassment to epidemiology, *Community Medicine 6*, 37–46.

Doll, R. and Hill, A. B. (1964) Mortality in relation to smoking: Ten years' observations of British doctors, *British Medical Journal 1*, 1399–410.

Fox, A. J. and Shewry, M. (1988) New longitudinal insights into relationships between unemployment and mortality, *Stress Medicine 4*, 11–19.

Kay, J. P. (1832) *The Moral and Physical Conditions of the Working Classes Employed in the Cotton Manufacture in Manchester*, London: James Ridgeway.

Lovell, A. (1987) In whose interest is access to medical records withheld?, *B. J. Obs. and Gyn. 94*, 609–11.

Macintyre, S. (1986) The patterning of health by social position in contemporary Britain: Directions for sociological research, *Soc. Sci. Med. 23*, 393–415.

McKeown, T. and Lowe, C. R. (1966) *An Introduction to Social Medicine*, Oxford: Blackwell.

McQueen, D. (1988) Ch. 1, in RUHBC, *Changing the Public Health*, London: John Wiley.

Martin, C. J., Platt, S. D. and Hunt, S. M. (1987) Housing conditions and ill-health, *British Medical Journal 294*, 1125–7.

Platt, S. D. and Kreitman, N. (1985) Parasuicide and unemployment among men in Edinburgh 1968–1982, *Psychological Medicine 15*, 113–23.

Rose, G. and Marmot, M. G. (1981) Social class and coronary heart disease, *British Heart Journal 45*, 13–19.

Rosen, G. (1958) *A History of Public Health*, New York: MD Publications.

Rush, D. and Cassano, P. (1983) Relationship of cigarette smoking and social class to birth weight and perinatal mortality among all births in Britain 5–11 April 1970, *Journal of Epidemiology and Community Health 37*, 249–55.

Simpson, W. J. (1957) A preliminary report on cigarette smoking and the incidence of prematurity, *American Journal of Obstetrics and Gynaecology 73*, 808–15.

Sterling, T. D. (1978) Does smoking kill workers or working kill smokers? *International Journal of Health Services 8*, 437–52.

Townsend, P. and Davidson, N. (1982) *Inequalities in Health: The Black Report*, London: Penguin.
Whitehead, M. (1987) *The Health Divide*, London: Health Education Council.
World Health Organisation (1978) *The Declaration of Alma Ata*, W.H.O.: Geneva.
World Health Organisation (1986) *Ottawa Charter for Health Promotion*, Health and Welfare, Canada.

Agendas for a New Public Health

2

FRANK BECHHOFER

INDIVIDUALS, POLITICS AND SOCIETY: A DILEMMA FOR PUBLIC HEALTH RESEARCH

A few months ago, I rashly agreed to give a very short paper at a conference on 'The University and the Wider Concept of Health'. The purpose of that conference was to discuss how universities might become involved in the World Health Organisation programme, Health for All by the Year 2000, which as you all know takes a view of health as something more than the absence of 'illth' and thus all the more difficult to achieve. I was then encouraged by the organisers of this conference 'Changing the Public Health' to develop what I had to say at somewhat greater length and once again, there being no fool like an old fool, I agreed. Let me then first give you some edited highlights from that previous piece. At the heart of my theme are age-old dilemmas which I suspect are especially sharp in research on public health. Are institutions of learning dispassionate and detached seekers after truth, or bodies passionately and indissolubly involved with the societies in which they are embedded?

My starting point was the succession of reports and studies concerned with health which have emphasised its close association with social factors and especially social inequality in its various forms. There is overwhelming evidence that health and illness, even in a narrow sense, are clearly patterned by social rather than individual factors. As we widen the definition of health, that association must become even stronger. It would require spectacles with a truly deep tint of rose to see the good life in poverty, unemployment, poor housing, stressful and dangerous work conditions, an unclean environment, and a lack of recreational and leisure facilities.

12

The dilemmas would be less acute if the factors leading to poor health were simply scattered randomly around the population. But of course the literature shows they are highly structured – above all by occupation and class; by region; and, in very complex ways, by gender.

A recognition, admittedly somewhat muted, of the role of structured inequality is at the heart of the Welfare State. In 1942 in the preface to the report bearing his name, Beveridge identified five great evils to be tackled in order to improve welfare, almost identical to health in the sense I am using it today. They were want, ignorance, idleness, squalor and disease. And they were to be tackled by social security, education, full employment, building and environmental programmes and, of course, the National Health Service.

The Beveridge Report is 45 years behind us. We have made some progress since 1942 but all the data suggest that inequality has not been reduced and may indeed have increased. There are between 2.5 and 4 million unemployed depending on how you count them, low-income families abound, income is unevenly distributed and wealth even more so, vast tracts of housing are effectively uninhabitable, and homelessness is anything but uncommon. All these structural factors are closely related to health and illness. Of course the lot of the median person or family, indeed the bulk of the population, has improved but the range of inequality has not been reduced. And this suggests that a sizeable measure of redistribution would have a greater effect on health than anything short of an improbably large general increase in available resources of all kinds.

Unlike my previous audience, you will hardly need reminding that all class theorists, Marxist or Weberian, agree that inequality results to a greater or lesser degree from class processes, and that these are in turn an aspect of the distribution of power in a society. That, it is argued, is why structured inequality is so durable; the interests of structured groups of actors and institutions are involved and redistribution is successfully resisted, or indeed never reaches the political agenda. And those of you who are intellectual or conscientious objectors where class theory is concerned, may care to consider regional disparities. Whatever explanation you give, the regional variations in health and health provision are undeniable. Again, unless additional resources can be made available on a scale never before considered, redistribution will be necessary and I at least can see reasons why a shift from (say) the south-east of England to the north-west of England or, perish the thought, to the west of Scotland might meet opposition. These issues, then, are highly politicised, and politicised in a peculiarly explosive way. To summarise crudely, what I want you to take from my earlier argument is that social inequality is immensely important in matters of health, that it is systematically patterned by social rather than individual factors, that it would require considerable redistribution to make much impact, and that this is a very hot political potato.

Let me at this juncture emphasise a most important point. I am not trying to set up a false contest between the social and the individual, between sociologistic and psychologistic explanations. I have lived for the past 27 years in extremely close proximity to (and usually harmony with) a psychologist and I know better than to do any such thing. Individual actions do affect health and individuals can, sometimes, be persuaded to act in ways which improve their health or, at least, damage it less. Nor am I necessarily suggesting that the social factors are more important; it is an empirical issue, albeit not one which is easy to resolve, whether individual decisions about, say, smoking are more of a public health problem than poor housing conditions. And the question is even harder to resolve if you recall that my interest is in health in the widest sense rather than the absence of illness. We have no easy metric which enables us to balance a 60- or 70-year lifetime of poverty and poor housing conditions against 45 years of a relatively pleasant life brought to a nasty end by lung cancer.

The individual and the social are hard to disentangle for another reason. You would of course expect a sociologist to insist that what is at one level an individual issue is at another a social structural or political problem. But I suspect that you will not need much persuading that this *is* often the case. Decisions to smoke or not to smoke, to drink excessively, sensibly or not at all, are undoubtedly at one level purely individual decisions. But it is a very long time since Durkheim argued that even that most individual of acts, suicide, was socially structured. I would take a great deal of convincing that social factors do not have a great influence on those individual decisions which affect the health not only of the person concerned but often their families and sometimes others. Nor is it an earth-shattering novelty to claim that these are political minefields. Is it unduly cynical to believe that the tobacco companies (for instance) form a powerful political lobby, or that pollution might be more easily reduced if many of the major polluters were not concerned for their profits, or that successive Chancellors of the Exchequer have been very willing to receive income from tobacco or alcohol and generally unwilling for reasons both of finance and of political popularity to raise excise duties too sharply? These social and political forces set the scene within which individual choices are made.

Far from wishing to deny the importance of individual, psychological factors in health, it is central to what follows that they are important and that much interesting research deals with them. It is in principle possible to change the public health *both* by altering individual behaviours, which may or may not involve social or political intervention, *and* by altering the social environment. Individual and social explanations are not by and large mutually exclusive and they can lead to intervention at both an individual and a social level. What I wish you to bear in mind, however, is that they *can* be perceived as alternatives, and one kind of intervention can be preferred over the other because one kind of explanation appeals more than the other for intellectual, social or ideological reasons.

The next proposition I wish to put to you is that in any society at a particular point in time greater or lesser importance may be attached to the individual or to the structural, to the individual as determining his or her own fate, or the individual as affected by societal forces. In Western culture the person on the proverbial Clapham omnibus always *tends* to think in terms of individual explanations, something which will be familiar to any sociologist who has taught an introductory course, or discussed the causes of football hooliganism, domestic violence or the invention of a better mousetrap with anyone who is prepared to listen. This conviction frequently co-exists with a feeling that 'someone' – usually government – 'should do something about it'. This 'something' however is often in the form of action at the individual level – be it to stop vandalism, provide better child-care, or stop the brain drain of mousetrap inventors.

A strong individualistic ethos lies at the heart of all advanced capitalist societies and forms the baseline, as it were, around which variations occur. At the same time, to be sure, the general public are strongly in favour of certain kinds of collective provision; in Britain, for instance, the Health Service. The wide variation of attitudes and opinions, often held in what may appear to be inconsistent patterns, enables political parties and pressure groups, at both national and local level, to place somewhat greater emphasis either on the individual or the social, to couch their proposals in terms of individual effort or social responsibility.

To some extent all this is a matter of rhetoric and the swings from one position to another are probably less extreme than it seems at the time, but I further want to suggest to you that in many of the countries of the capitalist West and certainly in Britain, the emphasis is currently very heavily on the individual and the need for individual responsibility. An interesting, if controversial, example is provided by the very recent AIDS-prevention television advertisement focusing on the sharing of needles by drug users. The advertisement is clearly premised on the assumption that the decision to share or not to share needles is an individual one. If the user decides not to share, he or she will be able, somehow, to carry through that decision and, more important, it is up to them to work out how to do so. Another example in the news is the unrest in Scottish prisons. It seems a safe guess that the causes are multiple and complex, but the explanation immediately invoked by many involved, including the Secretary of State, is individual (i.e. that the problems are caused by 'a few hard men').

In brief, the red-hot political potato of social inequality and health exists side by side with, to mix metaphors, the more graspable nettle of the impact of individual behaviours.

All this seems to me to highlight three problem areas for social research generally which are especially acute for public health research. These are the choice of research topic and funding; the carrying through of research findings into action; and a number of problems of research strategy. My remarks refer primarily to the British situation which I know best but I am pretty certain they are of wider application.

There is no simple relationship between what academics want to research, what the powerful would like researched (or not), and what gets funded by research councils, trusts and foundations or companies. But at the margins, some things are easier to finance than others; some issues appeal while others do not. It may be the case that some projects are more acceptable to those who hold the purse strings than others. What is certain is that researchers believe this is so. It is a safe bet that research has not been done in some sensitive research settings because access has never been sought rather than because access has been denied.

I hope it is clear by now that the choice is not between good and bad, worthwhile and puerile research but between pairs of respectable and defensible alternatives. Several processes then combine to encourage certain kinds of research at the expense of others.

Research Councils are becoming increasingly *dirigiste*, putting more of their research income into initiatives defined by the Council and less into projects proposed by researchers. In proposing these initiatives they have half an eye on the ABRC and at least a fraction of an eye on their paymasters. Even if research topics are not chosen because of their political respectability they are presented in the most politically acceptable way.

Because a great deal of research is now being done by large research teams, many of whom are on short-term contracts, the problems of continuity of financing weigh very heavily on researchers, leaders of research teams and directors of research centres. Furthermore the great time pressures under which people work lead them to submit grant applications at the last moment, a problem exacerbated by the infrequent (and inconsistent) deadlines laid down by different funding agencies. As a result there is usually insufficient time for two bites at the cherry. The consequences of a grant application being turned down encourage the choice of the safer of two or several alternatives.

Researchers are increasingly turning to commercial companies to augment what is available from the public arena. Often this research is carried out under acceptable terms of non-interference and rights to publication. But it is likely that there is an effect on the setting of the research agenda; certain topics are more likely to appeal or be financed in the first instance than others.

A large research project would be required to test my proposition that all this leads to rather more reaching for the graspable nettle than juggling with hot potatoes.

Even if you are sceptical, I suspect you will assent more readily to the notion, albeit still unresearched, that when it comes to the application of research findings, proposals to amend individual behaviour find more favour than proposals to alter the social environment. In many societies at the present time, but especially here in Britain, the amount of real change effected by the radical right is open to question, but it is I think undeniable that they have had an influence in the realm of ideas. Individualism and self-help are to be encouraged, the good life for all will result from a much larger cake rather than more equal slices, and the larger cake will be more easily baked if there are fewer restraints on ingredients or cooking methods. I must emphasise that I am not making a party political point here; whether all this rhetoric is to your taste or whether it sticks in your craw as it does in mine is not to the point. The prevailing climate favours certain social explanations at the expense of others; action suggested by some kinds of research is more likely to be adopted. To the extent that researchers, in our case today in the public health field, want their findings to be taken seriously and to lead to action, they are going to find it difficult to avoid the research agenda being set in particular ways, the findings of particular projects being taken up more readily than others, and their consultancy and evaluation services being sought for one kind of programme rather than another.

All this raises serious problems of the best route forward. Public health is after all concerned with fundamental issues – who lives and dies and why, the quality of life or death, programmes to effect change. Because of this should one, to return to my mixed metaphors, be running against the tide with a hot potato? If successful the gains might be enormous but there has to be a serious risk of achieving nothing. Or should one, donning gloves against contamination, go for the more graspable nettle even if one suspects, as I do, that the gains are likely to be relatively small?

Secondly, it is in the nature of our trade and the institutions in which we work to see everything as an educational or research problem. This predisposes us to sympathise with the twin arguments that people can be educated towards better health and that we need to understand the social processes involved in public health better if we are to act rationally and successfully. Is there then a risk that we shall bury our heads in the sand? The evidence that social inequality affects health in the widest sense is pretty inescapable. Do we really need a great deal more research to convince ourselves that Beveridge's five great evils of want, ignorance, idleness, squalor and disease are extremely unlikely to be good for us or that, while there are escape routes from these evils for individuals as a result of individual action, something more is needed if they are to become less rigidly socially structured?

Thirdly we should perhaps examine a little more closely the academic fear of 'being political'. I do not wish to get into a debate on value-freedom but let me at least say briefly that like Weber I am for it, if much more sceptical about its achievability! I am not arguing for a Marxist position of praxis. But as Stephen Lukes pointed out years ago, there is the third face of power. We should beware of setting the agenda in such a way that only the anodyne is defined as non-political and political comes to be equated with the unpalatable. In other words, research of the highest technical standards, as objective as research can ever be, may be defined as 'political' if it comes to unpopular conclusions, or seems to point inexorably in certain policy directions. This can occur in societies of all political hues and can be dealt with in different ways. In some societies it leads to harsh repression be it of the left or the right. In others it will be made explicitly clear that certain topics are off limits and not to be researched. In our society it is more likely that it will prove difficult to get funds, or access, and if the research is carried out, that it will be quietly buried and forgotten. The challenge which all social researchers face, and public health researchers face acutely, is how one responds to that situation.

I conclude with three quotes:

> The quality and duration of life are social variables which have always depended upon an almost infinite range of economic and social factors, the most important of which in modern times are levels of real income, the degree of adulteration of food, the quantity and quality of housing, sanitation, paving, sewerage, water supply, open spaces, working conditions and the public supply of the basic social services, of which education stands at the head of the list.

> Few subjects so easily spark off the flames of controversy as the question of the role of the state in economic and social development.

> The question of the extent of state intervention depends largely on the willingness of the economically wealthy and powerful groups to tax themselves, to reduce their incomes by restrictive legislation or to restrict their freedom of social, economic or political action.

I hope you will agree that this summarises many of the issues I have raised and chimes well with what I understand is known as the new public health. It is then perhaps sobering to contemplate that the quotes come from the introduction written by that great social historian, Michael Flinn, to the Edinburgh University Press reprint of Edwin Chadwick's, *The Sanitary Condition of the Labouring Population of Great Britain,* first published in 1842.

3

DAVID BLANE

PREVENTIVE MEDICINE AND PUBLIC HEALTH: ENGLAND AND WALES 1870–1914

Introduction

This paper is a preliminary examination of the contribution of preventive medicine to the improvement in the health of the population of England and Wales during the period 1870–1914. By preventive medicine is meant both the efforts of those such as the sanitary reformers who wished to change the population's material conditions of existence and the advice about a 'healthy lifestyle' which was offered by the medical profession and by the fore-runners of the health visitor and social work professions. The years 1870–1914 were chosen for study because during these years the mortality rates fell more dramatically than in any other period since the introduction in 1837 of the reliable recording of death. The paper draws heavily on F. B. Smith's encyclopaedic study of medical issues during this period (Smith 1979) and in particular its detailed descriptions of what we would now call preventive medicine and health education.

The purpose of this paper is to suggest, in the light of events during 1870–1914, what might be the most effective preventive strategies today. This is an inherently hazardous undertaking, because the 'lessons of history' always need to be interpreted in context, but an historical perspective nevertheless remains useful.

Health improvements

To the extent that mortality rates can be seen as an indicator of a population's health, one can say that the health of the population of

England and Wales improved dramatically between 1870 and 1914. The mortality rate of the 25–35 years age group, for example, fell in an approximately linear fashion from 9.6 per thousand in 1870 to 4.4 per thousand in 1914, and the mortality rates of most other age groups fell by a similar 50 per cent during this period. The exceptions to this general pattern were the 0–5 years and the age groups over 45 years, whose mortality rates were relatively stable from 1870 to 1900, and only started to fall after that date (Registrar General 1921).

It is important to bear in mind that this improvement started from a very low base line. It is possible to obtain some idea of this baseline by recalling that some 40 per cent of young men were, at the *end* of this improvement, still judged as physically unfit for military service in World War I (Oddy 1982), and it is likely that the proportion who were physically unfit was greater in the other, normally less healthy age groups. The level of morbidity *before* the 1870–1914 improvement, then, must indeed have been high.

Prevention

Prevention during this period can be divided into health education and preventive reforms; the former deriving from the medical profession and the fore-runners of the health visiting and social work professions, and the latter being implemented through local and central government. These two strategies will be considered separately, although of course some individuals were members of both groups.

Confronted by the living conditions which were endured by a large proportion of the urban working class, it must have been difficult for health educators to decide where to start. Smith, for example, described a study of infant diarrhoea deaths by the MOH for Bradford in 1878 in which such deaths were found to be more frequent where the excreta bucket, between its daily emptying, was kept under the food shelf. Although this practice emerged as the cause of the 'excess' mortality, the 'normal', though extremely high mortality rate was presumably due to the absence of piped water, the lack of cooking facilities and the overcrowding which were noted but then ignored. This study exemplifies the general approach to health education which emerges from Smith's book. Professional advice concentrated on people's behaviour and pushed into the background the material context which encouraged such behaviour. The link between dirt, parental neglect and infant mortality was emphasised, for example, while the poverty in which all three flourished was ignored. This apparently was seen as realistic, because the causes identified were conceivably remediable within the existing status quo; a position which was reinforced by the dominant miasma theory's stress on cleanliness.

The same framework ensured that drug consumption would also be a subject of health advice. In 1904, for example, Sir John Gorst argued in the House of Commons that the nation's poor health was partly due to juvenile smoking and the consumption of stewed tea. Equally under attack was the near universal consumption of alcohol, and the enjoyment of opium which was popular in industrial areas as well as the Fen country. The consumption of these drugs should be discouraged, it was argued, both because of their direct ill-effects and because their purchase meant less money for necessities.

Much health education was directed at women, particularly in relation to reproduction and child-rearing. The medical profession was so opposed to contraception that it rarely discussed the issue, although the occasional exception clearly revealed its attitude. The Lancet, for example, replied to an advocate of contraception that 'The expedients recommended for preventing conception are as injurious to morals and to health as they are physically loathsome and repulsive'. The profession also considered female employment to be a major cause of the high infant mortality rate, and saw the relationship as mediated through artificial feeding, neglect and the use of opium-based sedatives. Dr. McMillan, for example, argued in 1885 that '. . . women in modern society sought employment and resorted to bottle feeding to free themselves from what ought to be their first duty'. This concern that women should devote themselves to producing and raising many healthy children was partly motivated by patriotism. Sir John Gorst, in the speech referred to earlier, argued that women '. . . in limiting their offspring were careless of their duty to the Empire'. Similarly Dr. Ewart, in the Lancet debate also referred to above, stated: 'Love of offspring is the healthiest sign of a race, and the natural strength which is its reward stands revealed in connection with armaments and now more than ever in connection with colonising power'. Indeed so wedded to this position was the profession that it opposed pasteurisation of milk partly on the grounds that it '. . . made it easy for mothers to avoid breast-feeding and careful motherhood'. As such quotations suggest, what is now called victim-blaming was never far from the profession's thinking. 'Lazy, drunken and shiftless mothers' might be blamed for poor child health, and many accepted that '. . . the poor's death rate was not due to poverty, but rather to their ignorance, intemperance and improvidence'.

Such analyses, however, rarely led to detailed studies or proposed solutions.

In contrast to such comforting rationalisations was the health-visiting movement's assiduous work and sensible advice about infant management. This was probably the most successful part of health education during the period, even though it experienced considerable problems. Doctors were often unco-operative, sometimes offensive, and became angry if private patients were visited. In addition, the poor who perhaps needed their help most were frequently hostile. This hostility was not groundless: the poor were often unable to afford the carbolic, soap, milk and whitewash which the visitors recommended, and their constrained lives had great difficulty in adopting the routines which the visitors advocated. Nevertheless, the health visitors persevered, and in the process educated generations of mothers, as well as the medical profession, in the basics of infant hygiene, feeding and growth and development.

While the record of health education during this period was, with the exception of health visiting, not particularly distinguished, preventive reforms achieved perhaps their greatest successes. These reforms need to be seen in context, however, because they interacted with the rise in real wages which will be discussed in the next section. For the moment the point can be illustrated by the legislation against the sale of diseased meat and the adulteration of bread and milk. The relevant by-laws tended to be passed and, more importantly, enforced only when workers could afford better quality goods as the result of their increased real wages.

It was, however, in the area of clean water, hygienic disposal of sewage, drainage and clean, paved streets that the preventive reforms had their greatest success. Most of the relevant Acts were enabling legislation, which allowed local authorities to determine the timing and pace with which the improvements were introduced. Opposition to the reforms was common; rate-payers were often deterred by the cost, while the unenfranchised objected to the financing and pricing arrangements. As a result, while most of the wealthier areas of most towns had been improved by 1870, the conditions of the majority were little changed. By the 1880s, however, working class attitudes began to change in favour of the reforms, and the 'improvements' continued their slow spread. The speed of this spread should not be exaggerated, and it was not until the early years of the twentieth century that the domestic water supply in Britain became safe, uninterrupted and near-universal. In Smith's words it was not until, say 1905 that '. . . the greater accessibility of safe water and food had for the first time made the pursuit of health rationally possible' for much of the working class.

Living standard

As we have seen, the sanitary reforms were implemented locality by locality over a period of decades. Because these reforms were locally financed, the timing of their introduction was greatly influenced by the wealth of the local population, and the spread of the reforms in the late nineteenth century reflected a growth in general affluence. This growing affluence needs to be examined both because it was the material basis of the preventive reforms and for its wider role in the aetiological process.

Perhaps the best available measure of 'general affluence' during this period is real wages; that is, money wages in relation to prices, or how much wages can buy. Before examining how real wages changed between 1870 and 1914, however, it is worth considering the weaknesses of this measure. Firstly, real wages ignore the living standards of those households which do not depend on wages. However, this is probably of minor importance for present purposes because some three-quarters of the population depended on wages during the period (Hobsbawm, 1968) and, given their higher mortality rates, families dependent on wages probably accounted for some 80 to 85 per cent of total mortality at each age-group. Secondly, real wages ignore '. . . the hours of work, the physical and social conditions of the workplace, the quality of housing, the means of meeting misfortunes such as sickness and unemployment, the prevailing level of health, the squalor and the amenities of the towns, as well as the number of dependents in the household' (Phelps-Brown and Browne 1968). This is an important point because, as we will see, some of the things on which workers spent their increased real wages were, at first sight, not commodities. Finally, real wages reflect the living standards of only that section of the workforce which is in paid employment, and therefore this measure has to be seen in relation to unemployment levels and the business cycle. It has been argued elsewhere that apparent anomalies between mortality rates and real wages during the period 1870 to 1914 can be explained in this way (Blane 1988).

Bearing in mind these reservations, real wages rose by 66 per cent between 1870 and 1900, and were subsequently unchanged, in fact fell slightly, up to 1914 (Wood, 1909; Phelps-Brown and Browne 1968). Unemployment was high during the period of rising real wages (1873–1898 was known to contemporaries as 'The Great Depression'), and only fell when the economy

grew after 1900 (Mitchell and Deane 1962). During the period
1900–1914, therefore, although real wages were stationary, a
growing proportion of the working class was benefitting from this
much higher standard of living.

The effect of this rising standard of living on individuals was,
for most, mediated through the family structure, and during this
period the family was subjected to conflicting pressures. On the
one hand there were factors which lowered family income. The
married women's labour force participation rate, for example, fell
to an historic low of 10 per cent by 1900 (Hakim 1985), and the
1870 Education Act virtually eliminated child labour (Hobsbawm
1954). In contrast were factors which had the opposite effect.
Women's employment shifted from low paid home production,
such as ribbon and lace making, into better paid factory jobs, often
in the new food industries (Hobsbawm 1954). Similarly, the
practice of family planning spread, and the birth rate fell by more
than one-third between 1870 and 1914 (OPCS 1974). Although
these factors would have affected individual family incomes in
varying ways, their combined effect on general family incomes was
probably in balance. In other words, the rising real wages probably
indicate rising individual consumption.

The increased real wages were spent in a variety of ways. A large
proportion was individually spent on the purchase of commodities, particularly a more varied, less protein-deficient diet (Blane
1987). Some was collectively spent on, for example, the sanitary
reforms. Some was spent at work on Friendly Society subscriptions
which offered benefit during illness and unemployment, and finally
some was 'spent' at work in the form of shorter hours and a less
punishing work regime: 'The pressure for shorter hours had itself
been both permitted and instigated by the rise in real rates of pay,
and the same effect was seen in a reduction of effort by piece
workers who did not need to produce so much as before in order
to obtain a given real weekly wage' (Phelps-Brown and Browne
1968).

In summary, then, individual living standards rose by some two-
thirds between 1870 and 1914. The new wealth was spent in a variety
of ways, and as McKeown has shown (McKeown 1976, 1979), it
was this improvement in the standard of living which was primarily
responsible for the fall in mortality rates during these years.

Conclusions

It now remains to assess the contribution of preventive medicine
to the dramatic improvements which occurred in the health of the

population of England and Wales between 1870 and 1914, and to consider whether this experience suggests any lessons for preventive medicine today.

Certain similarities between these two periods are striking. Perhaps the most obvious of these are the concern about drug consumption and the tendency towards victim-blaming. The drug consumption which concerned preventive medicine in the earlier period, such as juvenile smoking, stewed tea, opium and alcohol, were primarily modified by legislation and perhaps also by a need for less powerful drugs once the quality of life had improved; in this respect at least, 'official advice' seems to have had little effect on individual choices. The tendency to blame a population's poor health on the ignorance and laziness of its members was similarly ineffective, although Smith draws attention to one important exception to this general rule. He argues that the early health visitor movement may have contributed to the fall in the infant mortality rate after 1900 by spreading knowledge about infant hygiene and feeding. He goes on to show, however, that this health education was effective only because the hygiene infrastructure was more or less in place by 1900 and the campaign was pursued in an organised and systematic way by an increasingly specialised proto-professional group.

The most spectacular health education failure of the period, in contrast, found women increasingly doing the opposite of official advice. First, family planning and contraception became ever more popular, despite these practices being branded as unpatriotic and unnatural, and second, after 1900, married women once again started to rejoin the workforce, although the poor health of infants and young children had been long blamed on their neglect by working mothers. In this instance, at least, lay behaviour was probably more sensible than preventive medicine because the combination of fewer children and the wife/mother's wages would have helped to ensure that the standard of living of individual family members was capable of sustaining health.

Underlying these failures was preventive medicine's concern to be 'realistic' and its consequent emphasis on factors which were seen as remediable within the existing status quo. Instead of an objective account of the factors which underlay the population's poor health, preventive medicine tacitly ignored those factors which failed this test of political acceptability. The emphasis was on how people should change their behaviour within existing conditions, rather than on how existing conditions should be changed. The sanitary reforms represented the limits of this approach, because they both threatened the interests of the private water industry and involved large-scale investment by local authorities. The gradual spread of the sanitary reforms was due to the perseverance and political skills of their advocates and to the growing affluence of local populations, and it is tempting to see the coincidence of interests between laymen and experts as underlying this success, with expert comment having sharpened lay perceptions of their own squalor, thus ensuring that it would be rectified as soon as this was financially possible.

A similar coincidence of interests, however, was lacking over many other issues. As we have seen, the importance which laymen gave to improved nutrition and shorter working hours did not reflect the low priority which preventive medicine had given to these issues. Once again, it seems that the lay population was more sensible than the experts because, as McKeown and Lowe (1966) have shown, the bulk of the fall in mortality during this period resulted from a reduction in deaths due to air-borne infections; these could not have been affected by the sanitary reforms, but would have responded to improved immunity as the result of better nutrition and less chronic exhaustion.

On balance, then, the effect of preventive medicine was mixed. It seems to have been least effective where it addressed itself to individuals and urged them to change their behaviour in ways which either they did not want or they perceived, often correctly, as not being in their own best interests. In contrast, preventive medicine was most successful when it sharpened the perceptions of already felt needs and organised collective solutions to them. Underlying both the successes and failures, however, was an approach which ensured that the most important preventive health measures were taken without preventive medicine being significantly involved.

This need not have happened. The improvement in living standards, which was primarily responsible for the improvement in health, was neither automatic nor evenly spread. Rather, it was won through myriad local struggles over a variety of issues, such as wages and hours of work, and although better health was never a demand in these struggles, this was a medically predictable consequence of their success. Preventive medicine could have related to these struggles as successfully as it fought for the sanitary reforms, but was prevented from doing so by its political 'realism' and, one suspects, its desire for respectability.

This analysis suggest that preventive medicine, to be effective, should start from the lay population's felt needs, investigating the health consequences of these and helping to organise a response to them. There has always been a minority within preventive medicine which has adopted this approach; it would be interesting to know why the majority does not join them.

References

Blane, D. (1987). The value of labour power and health, in G. Scambler, (ed). *Sociological Theory and Medical Sociology*, London: Tavistock Publications.

Blane, D. (1988). Real wages, the economic cycle and mortality: England and Wales 1870–1914 (in press).

Hakim, C. (1985). Social monitors: population censuses as social surveys, in M. Blumer (ed.) *Essays on the History of British Sociological Research*, Cambridge: Cambridge University Press.

Hobsbawm, E. J. (1954) The labour aristocracy in 19th century Britain, in J. Saville (ed). *Democracy and the Labour Movement*, London: McMillan.

Hobsbawm, E. J. (1968) *Industry and Empire*, Harmondsworth: Penguin.

McKeown, T. (1976) *The Modern Rise of Population*, London: Edward Arnold.

— (1979) *The Role of Medicine*, Oxford: Blackwell.

McKeown, T. and Lowe, C. R. (1966) *An Introduction to Social Medicine*, Oxford: Blackwell.

Mitchell, B. R. and Deane, P. (1962) *Abstract of British Historical Statistics*, Cambridge: Cambridge University Press.

Oddy, D. J. (1970) Working-class diets in late nineteenth-century Britain, *Economic History Review 23*, 314–22.

— (1982) The health of the people, in T. Barker and M. Drake (eds) *Population and Society in Britain 1850–1980*, London: Batsford.

OPCS (Office of Population Censuses and Surveys) (1974) *Birth Statistics (England and Wales)*, Series no. 1, London: HMSO.

Phelps-Brown, E. H. and Browne, M. H. (1968) *A Century of Pay*, New York: St Martin's Press.

Registrar General's Statistical Review of England and Wales (1921) No.1, London: HMSO.

Smith, F. B.(1979) *The People's Health 1830–1910*, London: Croom Helm.

Wood, G. H. (1909) Real wages and the standard of comfort since 1850, *Journal of Royal Statistical Society*, 72, 91–103.

4

ALEX SCOTT-SAMUEL

BUILDING THE NEW PUBLIC HEALTH:
A PUBLIC HEALTH ALLIANCE AND A
NEW SOCIAL EPIDEMIOLOGY

Introduction: The New Public Health

The first part of this paper is concerned with the development in the United Kingdom (UK) of what is generally known as the New Public Health Movement, and in particular of the Public Health Alliance. The second part deals with the need to develop a new social epidemiology in order to provide an adequate theoretical framework for the new public health.

In the UK the background to the development of the new public health was the structural reorganisation of the National Health Service (NHS) in 1974. One result of this reorganisation was the loss of the old public health framework whereby publicly accountable Medical Officers of Health (MOH) were employed by local authorities to oversee the public health of the locality. While this was by no means ideal, it was at least the case that the MOH's role was seen as one of public health advocacy. In the years since 1974 the loss of this role, as a result of the Medical Officers of Health being absorbed into the Health Authorities of the NHS as community physicians, has caused an increasing amount of disquiet. In the 1970s this disquiet was perhaps most clearly voiced in the publications of the Unit for the Study of Health Policy in the Department of Community Medicine at Guy's Hospital. In a series of publications (Draper, Best and Dennis, 1976; Unit for the Study of Health Policy, 1978; Unit for the Study of Health Policy, 1979) the current state of public health in Britain was outlined and an ecological model was proposed, within which community

29

physicians could once again contribute to public health promotion. 'Rethinking Community Medicine' introduced the concept of the Health Promotion Team and was effectively the forerunner of the current fashion for health promotion in the UK – though the model which it described was very much more enterprising than the version currently in vogue.

Around the same time a different aspect of the new public health was getting off the ground. In 1977 the first Community Health Projects were established in the UK; these now form one aspect of an estimated 12,000 UK community health initiatives (Watt, 1986; Community Health Initiatives Resource Unit and London Community Health Resource, 1987). Community health projects are essentially concerned with lay community workers, usually in deprived areas of towns and cities, who take an approach which starts from the social origins of much ill-health. They tend to be concerned with providing support, education, awareness raising and campaigning on health issues in the neighbourhood.

The Black Report on inequalities in health (Townsend and Davidson, 1988) has also been influential, both in making people aware that the substantial and increasing social inequalities in health dictate the need for a new public health movement, and in itself giving rise to local Black reports in a number of areas of the UK (Croxteth Area Working Party, 1983; Townsend, Simpson and Tibbs, 1985; Manchester Joint Consultative Committee (Health), 1985; Betts, 1985; Ginnety, Kelly and Black, 1985; Thunhurst, 1985; Appleby, 1986).

At the level of public policy the influence of the World Health Organisation (WHO) in the 1980s has also been substantial. The publication in 1978 of the Declaration of Alma Ata (World Health Organisation, 1978) and the subsequent development of the WHO strategy for 'Health For All by The Year 2000' effectively set an agenda for the new public health in Europe. The WHO Targets for Health For All (WHO, 1985) which were endorsed by the British Government, have provided the impetus for a number of conferences and publications on the theme of healthy public policy (Kings Fund Institute 1987; WHO, Health and Welfare Canada, Canadian Public Health Association 1986; WHO, 1987a; Robbins, 1987; Healthy Cities Intersectoral Committee, 1988). Also very influential in this area has been the germinal work of Milio (1981).

There has also been a parallel development within local authorities of activities relating to the new public health. Many local authorities, as well as undertaking local Black reports have formed

ALTERNATIVE STRATEGIES FOR PREVENTION

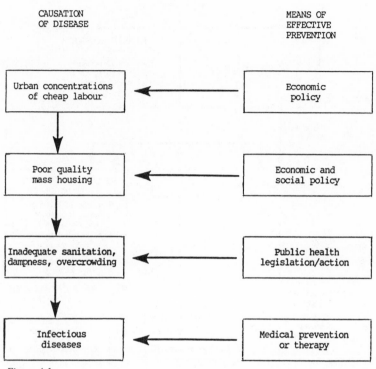

CAUSATION
OF DISEASE

MEANS OF
EFFECTIVE
PREVENTION

Urban concentrations of cheap labour	◄	Economic policy
Poor quality mass housing	◄	Economic and social policy
Inadequate sanitation, dampness, overcrowding	◄	Public health legislation/action
Infectious diseases	◄	Medical prevention or therapy

Figure 4.1

new health committees, have employed full-time health officers and have been active in promoting the public health in their role as service providers (Rayner and Moran, 1987; Health Education Authority and Oxford City Council, 1987).

Figure 1 exemplifies the model on which the new public health is based. An epidemiological chain of causation resulting in ill-health is shown in the left-hand column. The conventional response within the medical model (shown in the bottom right-hand box) is to await the development of ill-health and then to treat it with medical means such as drugs, surgery or radiotherapy; at best a medicalised preventive approach is taken which involves attempting to prevent ill-health through individualistic medical means, such as immunisation or screening. The public health model, however,

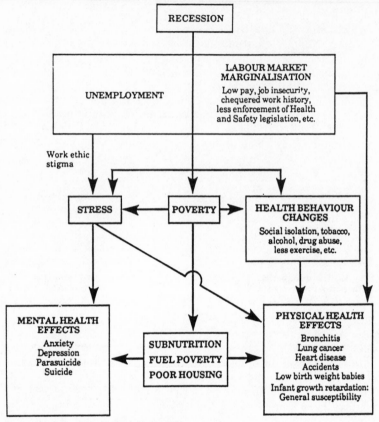

Unemployment and Health Study Group, 1986

Figure 4.2

seeks to prevent ill-health occurring in the first place by means of action at the level of public policy. This is shown more clearly in Figure 2, which demonstrates the complex set of relationships underlying the ill-health resulting from recession and unemployment (Unemployment and Health Study Group, 1986). While there are a number of points at which intervention can prevent ill-health, what is clear is that virtually all of these points relate to action at the level of social or economic policy, be it in terms of job creation, destigmatising the status of the unemployed, or taking action to alleviate fuel poverty.

During the last 2 years there has been a flood of reports on health inequalities, many of them resulting from the discussions which followed the Black Report (Wilkinson, 1986; Heartbeat Wales, 1987; Whitehead, 1988; BMA Board of Science and Education, 1987; Health Promotion Research Trust, 1987; National Children's Bureau, 1987; Radical Statistics Health Group, 1987; Townsend, Phillimore and Beattie, 1987). In addition there have been many publications on single aspects of the new public health such as unemployment (Smith, 1987), women's health (Orr, 1987) and the health of racial minorities (McNaught, 1987).

The extent to which the new public health has established itself is reflected in the recent review of the specialty of community medicine in England, by a committee chaired by the Chief Medical Officer of the English Department of Health, Sir Donald Acheson (Committee of Enquiry, 1988). This report actually proposes the renaming of the specialty of community medicine to 'public health medicine'. As with the new Health Promotion, what emerges is likely to be a pale shadow of the plans of its originators. (Anonymous, 1988; Ashton, 1988), but this is none the less an indication of the hold that the public health concept has gained in a relatively short space of time.

The Public Health Alliance

The chief reason for the renewed interest in public health, by local authorities and pressure groups has been the visible deterioration in many of the areas that influence people's health. As income differentials between rich and poor have widened in the 1980s, there have been major reductions in the building of houses, massive increases in long-term unemployment, and cuts in education, the NHS and other public services. The effect on people's health has been all too apparent (Whitehead, 1988). The result has been an increasing awareness and concern about the public health as a general issue. This concern led to the formation in 1986 and the public launch in July 1987, of a new policy and pressure group concerned with promoting the public health in all its aspects – the Public Health Alliance (Smith, 1986; Anonymous, 1987; Scott-Samuel, 1987). The aim of the Public Health Alliance (PHA) is to bring together voluntary and community groups, professional associations, local authorities, trade unions and individuals to promote and defend the public health in the UK. In focusing on the full breadth of public health issues, the approach of the PHA echoes that of WHO in its strategy of 'Health For All by the Year 2000'.

The PHA is pursuing its aims in four main ways:

1.The provision of a national focus for stimulating and discussing health promoting activities in the UK.

2.The identification and strengthening of existing coalitions and the initiation of new ones to promote the public health.

3.The provision of resources to support research and action in public health promotion.

4.The undertaking of policy development, research and practical public health activities and the widespread publication of such work.

As an initial way of drawing attention to the aims of the PHA, a Charter for Health has been produced (PHA, 1987). The Charter takes a human rights approach to health and sets out the following as the essential basis of every citizen's right to good health:

Income which provides the material means to remain healthy.

Homes that are safe, warm, dry, secure and affordable.

Food that is safe, nourishing, widely available and cheap.

Transport that permits accessible safe travel at reasonable cost and encourages fuel economy and a clean environment.

Work that is properly rewarded, in or out of the home, which is worthwhile and free from hazards to health and safety.

Environments protected from dangerous pollution and radiation and planned to preserve and enhance our quality of life.

Public services which provide care for those who need it and support for carers; clean safe water and waste disposal, adequate child-care and recreational facilities.

Education and health promotion which give all the necessary information to keep us healthy and the confidence and resources to tackle the causes of ill-health.

Comprehensive health services, properly resourced, free at the point of use and sensitive to our health needs.

Equal opportunity to good health regardless of class, race, sex, physical ability, age, or sexual orientation.

The PHA has established its initial base in Birmingham and is currently producing a formal constitution. A number of action groups have been established which are busily producing and publishing discussion papers on the major public health themes of the day.

The breadth of the PHA's remit is daunting and it will face the substantial and well established conflicts of interest between those who promote the public health and the institutional and

Areas of transformation	Principles of transformation		
	Status quo	Reclassification of present approaches	Definition of new approaches
Nature of health and illness	(i) Illness = disease = discrete episodic changes in organ systems (ii) Static "social factors" as disease determinants.	Reclassification of diseases on the basis of their social origins.	New health practice starting from subjective social meaning of illness.
Study of health and illness	(i) Expert scientific studies of disease entities. (ii) Expert scientific surveys of consumer experience and priorities.	(i) Expert individual studies of illness biography. (ii) Expert individual studies of social processes in the production of illness.	Collective community-based studies of health and illness production with appropriate use of experts as required.
Management of health and illness	Specialisation based on roles and skills; organ systems, age group or sex of patients.	(i) Reclassification of some technicians (e.g. doctors) into roles relating to the social origins of illness (ii) Reclassification of other health workers into community-based teams effectively acting as "composite community workers"	Deskilling of majority of health workers into the minimum necessary roles of (i) Generic community worker (ii) Health/social counsellor (iii) Technical backup force (mainly in hospitals).

Figure 4.3

commercial opposition. The PHA is declaring itself non-party political in its orientation; in the public health minefield, allies and antagonists can emerge from all quarters. Most importantly, the PHA has every intention of making a reality of the principles behind the WHO Health For All strategy; the reduction of inequalities, intersectoral collaboration, primary health care and above all, community participation. Given the virtual absence of any of these from the current public health arena, the outlook for the future of the PHA in promoting public health in the UK must be good.

Towards a social epidemiology

A week is a long time in politics, but a decade is nothing in public health policy. Despite the almost universal support for the materialist approach to health which was favoured in the Black Report, there has been very little development, in the years since its publication, towards a materialist epidemiology conceptually adequate to service the new public health. I shall outline some of the possibilities by reference to Figure 3 (Scott-Samuel, 1981), which illustrates the possibilities for transforming our understanding of the nature of health, the epidemiology with which we study it, and the health care systems with which we manage illness.

The new public health requires a new, truly social, truly critical, development in epidemiology to produce – and here I use R. D. Laing's definition of science (Laing, 1967) – '. . . a form of knowledge adequate to its subject'. The form of this epidemiology has yet to be fully defined, but it seems likely, given the nature of the new public health that, among the necessary criteria, it should be: participative; non-expertist; subjective; and collective in its nature. In the early 1980s the journal *Radical Community Medicine* published a number of papers aimed at establishing a debate around the development of such an epidemiology (Davies, 1982; Paterson, 1981; Jones, 1983). More recently, the World Health Organisation has begun to acknowledge the need for such developments, and its current discussions on Target 32 of the Health For All targets (which is concerned with research policy for Health For All), are very much relevant to this aim. A recent WHO statement on research policy for Health For All stated that 'the users of research findings and those who will be influenced by them have to be involved from the very beginning in deciding on research priorities and, so far as possible, in designing and conducting the studies' (WHO, 1987b). It is also instructive to quote from a recent publication by the WHO European Regional Officer for Maternal and Child Health: 'The people can be given the data on the services they use . . . they can ask us to give them technical assistance so that they can correctly define the problem, and collect and analyse the data, and then they can use the results as they see fit, to improve their own health and health-care . . . I believe we will see the emergence of a new epidemiology – community epidemiology – in which the people of a community do their own epidemiology with a little help from their friends: us' (Wagner, 1988).

Much of the momentum for a new social epidemiology is coming from social scientists, and the Changing the Public Health Conference exemplifies this (see, for example, the papers by Blane; Klesse and Sonntag; and Popay and Bartley).

In considering the new social epidemiology, it is helpful first to discuss our understanding of the health and illness which this epidemiology is to describe. The first row in Figure 3 begins by describing the status quo – in other words, the medical model of health viewed in terms of diseases in individuals. Inasmuch as the social origins of health are considered, it is in the form of static social factors (such as social class) being posited as determinants of disease. Even when this is done, the concern of present-day epidemiologists is more likely to be that of 'controlling out social factors' than of looking behind them to consider their nature.

A first move beyond a medical model might involve the reclassification of diseases on the basis of their social origins. One example of such an approach, with regard to legal and illegal drug use, is that taken by Cameron and Jones (1985):

> People use these drugs to treat a number of dis-eases including loneliness, shyness, sexual incompetence, social incompetence, ignorance, boredom, anxiety and depression. The causes of these dis-eases, indeed of all dis-ease, is a lack of harmony between the individual and the environment. This may be due to poverty, unemployment, bad working conditions, bad housing, overcrowding, or insufficient or unsuitable education or preparation to meet the crises of life. These dis-eases have, in themselves, components which are due to direct material processes and other components which are ideological. For example, the notion of sexual competence is largely subjective and feelings of adequacy or inadequacy are judged by the standards of the cinema, television or novels, or of the statements of friends and colleagues . . . We think that a major task for epidemiology in the immediate future is the study of the aetiology and classification of those dis-eases that provide a need for the drugs of solace, with the object of setting out a public programme for their prevention. (pp.21, 22, 27)

Another interesting and germinal piece of work in this field was published over 10 years ago by Draper, Best and Dennis (1977). This paper attempted a social taxonomy of diseases and states of ill-health, based upon their origins in the processes of production, distribution and consumption of resources within society. A further example of theoretical reformism within this field is Brownlea's concept of political epidemiology (Brownlea, 1981). However, the further transformation of such social concepts of health into a new formulation grounded in the subjective social meaning of health and illness is a development as yet untried.

We can now consider how these notions of a transformed understanding of health relate to the practice of epidemiology itself. At present, this can be loosely characterised (in the case of clinical epidemiology) in terms of expert scientific studies of disease entities. Present-day social epidemiology consists chiefly of expert scientific surveys of people's health experiences and priorities. Since moves away from expertist approaches to epidemiology are developing relatively slowly at present, reformism in this area is concerned primarily with the development of more subjective approaches – expert studies of illness from a biographical perspective – and with expert studies of social processes in the production of illness. Examples of the former include Cornwell's (1984) *Hard-Earned Lives: Accounts of Health and Illness from East London*:

> . . . in both public and private accounts the commonsense ideas and theories which govern the relationship people in the study have with health, illness and health services are grounded in their way of life . . . The private accounts of episodes of illness and the private aetiological theories showed that for people in the study there is no clear separation between illness and what is happening in the rest of their lives. The way in which they respond to feeling unwell is determined as much by their position in the sexual division of labour and at work as anything else, and they see illness as the product of the particular set of circumstances in which the person finds him or herself. This analysis has some practical implications for health education/promotion, and preventive health work. It suggests . . . that changes in commonsense ideas and theories about health and illness (and thus in health-related behaviour) are not likely to occur in the absence of changes in other areas of people's lives. It may therefore be more important to change people's position in relation to employment, for example, or to change the sexual division of labour, than constantly to direct attention to health attitudes and beliefs. (pp.205–6)

Graham (1984) is another researcher who has taken a biographical approach to health:

... story-telling counteracts the tendency of surveys to fracture women's experiences. As we've seen, social surveys encourage respondents to reduce their experiences to fragments which can be captured in a question-and-answer format. Stories, by contrast, provide a vehicle through which individuals can build up and communicate the complexity of their lives . . . stories are pre-eminently ways of relating individuals and events to social contexts, ways of weaving personal experiences into their social fabric. Moreover, stories provide a vehicle through which the existence and experience of inequality can be described. (p.119)

An early application of materialist epidemiology to the social production of illness was that of Dorn (1981). Like Cameron and Jones, he studied the use of drugs – in this case the use of alcohol by adolescents:

. . . local, social and economic structures (especially the labour market and the family) and also material conditions (such as housing, environment etc.) set the scene within which school leavers develop their various cultures . . . and within which drinking and other health-related behaviour occurs. . . . The social and economic relations obtaining within the family home vary, from area to area, in the degree to which they require teenage girls to work within the home, thus restricting their ability to compete equally in the labour market. In my study area, it was within the lower strata of the working class that the domestic commitments of teenage girls were greatest; these girls were generally expected to do a lot of domestic work, often looking after other members of the family, thus freeing the mother to do the waged work necessary to balance the family's budget. Such circumstances severely limit the ability of lower working class teenage girls to compete equally in the labour market, and to enter its service sector. These young female domestic workers do not have an economic independence to celebrate; they do not enter into mixed sex round-buying; in sharp contrast to service sector girls, they use flirtatious devices to obtain drinks from men. Their drinking practices reflect their acceptance of their social and economic position. (p.81)

Another recent example of a study of social process in the production of illness is Robinson's (1986) study of the association between hazardous work and low job security.

The ultimate aim of a transformed social epidemiology might be characterised in terms of collective, community-based studies of health and illness production, with appropriate use of experts as required. There have already been some moves in this direction, particularly in the Third World where the concept of participatory research has been developed in recent years, primarily under the aegis of adult education. Participatory research has been described as being composed of three inter-related processes (Society for Participatory Research in Asia, 1982):

    1. Collective investigation of problems and issues with the active participation of the constituency in the entire process.

    2. Collective analysis, in which the constituency develops a better understanding not only of the problems at hand but also of the underlying structural causes (socio-economic, political, cultural) of the problem.

    3. Collective action by the constituency aimed at long-term as well as short-term solutions to these problems. (p.2)

Additional criteria for participatory research (Hall, Etherington and Jackson, 1979) are:

    1. It should be action orientated.

    2. It should strengthen the voice of the powerless.

    3. It should be in and of itself of direct benefit to the community.

    4. It should reduce the dependence of the community on outside experts.

    5. It should make links between health issues and the broader social struggle for justice. (p.9)

All of these criteria are consistent with the WHO Health For All strategy and it will be interesting to see if links are made between the participatory research community and the developing WHO Research Strategy for Health For All. There is already in the UK the beginnings of a participatory research network which should assist in this process.

Much of the development of this kind of research in the health sector has been related to occcupational health and safety. In the UK, a recent example was a study of the effects on the health of bus drivers of the introduction of one-person operated buses (Joffe, Mackay and Mitchell, 1986). Two recent participatory studies in South Africa concern a respiratory survey related to a workplace pollutant (Health Information Centre, 1987) and a hearing loss survey related to noise at work (Technical Advice Group/National Union of Mineworkers Noise Group, 1987). There has also been established during the past two decades a tradition of participatory occupational epidemiology in Italy, which has been described in detail by Reich and Goldman (1984).

Although some recent developments in the UK give cause for optimism in this area (such as the Participatory Research Exchange and the Operational Research Society's new Community Operational Research Unit at Northern College), there is clearly a need for a central focus for the new social epidemiology – an institute in which the concepts, methods and practices outlined in this paper can be nurtured and fully developed.

References

Anonymous (1987) The Public Health Alliance, *Lancet 2*, 228.

Anonymous (1988) Back to the future – the reinvention of public health, (Editorial) *Lancet 1*,157–9.

Appleby, J. (1986) *Social Inequality and Public Health in Birmingham*, South Birmingham Health Authority.

Ashton, J. (1988) Acheson: a missed opportunity for the new public health, *BMJ 296*, 231–2

Betts, G. (1985) *Health in Glyndon*, London: Greenwich Health Rights Project

British Medical Association Board of Science and Education (1987) *Deprivation and Ill-Health*, London: British Medical Association.

Brownlea, A. (1981) From public health to political epidemiology, *Social Science and Medicine 15D*, 57–67.

Cameron, D. and Jones, I. (1985) An epidemiological and sociological analysis of the use of alcohol, tobacco and other drugs of solace, *Community Medicine 7*, 18–29.

Committee of Inquiry into the Future Development of the Public Health Function(1988) *Public Health in England*, London: HMSO.

Community Health Initiatives Resource Unit and London Community Health Resource (1987) *Guide to Community Health Projects*, London: CHIRU/LCHR.

Cornwell, J. (1984) *Hard-Earned Lives. Accounts of Health and Illness from East London*, London: Tavistock.

Croxteth Area Working Party (1983) *Report*. City Solicitor's Department, Liverpool City Council.

Davies, C. (1982) Criticising epidemiology :some notes on the debate, *Radical Community Medicine 11/12*, 6–15.

Dorn, N. (1981) Youth culture in the UK: independence and round drinking. Implications for health education, *International Journal of Health Education 24*, 77–82.

Draper, P. Best, G. and Dennis, J. (1976) *Health, Money and the National Health Service*, Unit for the Study of Health Policy, Dept. of Community Medicine, Guy's Hospital Medical School.

Draper, P. Best, G. and Dennis, J. (1977) Health and wealth, *Royal Society of Health Journal 97*, 121–6.

Ginnety, P. Kelly, K. and Black, M. (1985) *Moyard: a health profile*, Belfast: Eastern Health and Social Services Board.

Graham, H. (1984) Surveying through stories, in Bell, C. and Roberts, H. (eds.), *Social researching: Politics, Problems, Practice*, London: Routledge & Kegan Paul.

Hall, B. Etherington, A. and Jackson, T. (1979) *Evaluation, Participation and Community Health Care : Critique and Lessons*, Toronto: International Council for Adult Education.

Health Education Authority and Oxford City Council (1987) *Oxford _ a Healthy City Strategy*, London: HEA.

Health Information Centre (1987) Worker participation in a respiratory health survey, *Critical Health (Doornfontein, S.A.) 20*, 29–34.

Health Promotion Research Trust (1987) *The Health and Lifestyle Survey*, London: HPRT.

Healthy Cities Intersectoral Committee (1988) *The Liverpool Declaration on the Right to Health*, WHO Healthy Cities Project, Liverpool City Council.

Heartbeat Wales (1987) *Pulse of Wales Social Survey Supplement*, Cardiff: Heartbeat Wales.

Joffe, M. Mackay, T. and Mitchell, J. (1986) *Buswork and Health*, Birmingham: TURC Publishing.

Jones, I. (1983) A model of occupational health for community medicine, *Radical Community Medicine 14*, 28–31.

King's Fund Institute (1987) *Healthy Public Policy: a Role for the HEA*, London: KFI.

Laing, R. D. (1967) The politics of experience, in *The Politics of Experience and the Bird of Paradise*, Harmondsworth: Penguin

McNaught, A. (1987) *Health Action and Ethnic Minorities*, London: Bedford Square Press.

Manchester Joint Consultative Committee (Health) (1985) *Health Inequalities and Manchester*.

Milio, N. (1981) *Promoting Health Through Public Policy*, Philadelphia: F. A. Davis.

National Children's Bureau (1987) *Investing in the Future: Child health ten years after the Court Report*, London: NCB.

Orr, J. (ed.) (1987) *Women's Health in the Community*, Chichester: John Wiley & Sons.

Paterson, K. (1981) Theoretical perspectives in epidemiology – a critical appraisal, *Radical Community Medicine 8*, 21–9.

Public Health Alliance (1987) *A Charter For Public Health*, Birmingham: PHA (PO Box 1156, Kings Norton, Birmingham B30 2AZ).

Radical Statistics Health Group (1987) *Facing the Figures*, London: Radical Statistics.

Rayner, G. and Moran, G. (1987) Local Government and the

promotion of public health, in *Health Care UK 1987 – An Economic, Social and Policy Audit*, Hermitage: Policy Journals.

Reich, M. R. and Goldman, R. H. (1984) Italian occupational health: concepts, conflicts, implications, *American Journal of Public Health 74*, 1031–41.

Robbins, C. (ed.) (1987) *Health Promotion in North America: Implications for the UK*, Health Education Council and King Edward's Hospital Fund for London.

Robinson, J. (1986) Job hazards and job security, *Journal of Health Politics, Policy and Law 11*, 1–18.

Scott-Samuel, A. (1981) Towards a socialist epidemiology, *Radical Community Medicine 7*, 13–18.

Scott-Samuel, A. (1987) The Public Health Alliance, *THS Health Summary*, July/August, 6.

Smith, R. (1986) The need for a public health alliance, *BMJ 293*, 346–7.

Smith, R. (1987) *Unemployment and Health. A Disaster and a Challenge*, Oxford: Oxford University Press.

Society for Participatory Research in Asia (1982) *Participatory Research: An Introduction*, Toronto: International Council for Adult Education.

Technical Advice Group/National Union of Mineworkers Noise Group (1987) Organisational involvement in a noise-induced hearing loss survey, *Critical Health (Doornfontein, S.A.) 20*, 35–41.

Thunhurst, C. (1985) *Poverty and health in the City of Sheffield*, Environmental Health Department, Sheffield City Council.

Townsend, P. Simpson, D. and Tibbs, N. (1985) Inequalities in health in the City of Bristol: a preliminary review of statistical evidence, *International Journal of Health Services 15*, 637–63.

Townsend, P. Phillimore, P. and Beattie, A. (1987) *Deprivation and Health: Inequality and the North*, Beckenham: Croom Helm.

Townsend, P. and Davidson, N. (eds.) (1988) The Black Report, in *Inequalities in Health*, Harmondsworth: Penguin.

Unemployment and Health Study Group (1986) *Unemployment: A Challenge to Public Health*, Centre for Professional Development, Dept. of Community Medicine, University of Manchester.

Unit for the Study of Health Policy (1978) *The NHS in the Next 30 Years – a New Perspective on the Health of the British*, USHP, Dept. of Community Medicine, Guy's Hospital Medical School.

Unit for the Study of Health Policy (1979) *Rethinking Community Medicine: Towards a Renaissance in Public Health?* USHP, Dept. of Community Medicine, Guy's Hospital Medical School.

Wagner, M. (1988) Whose data is it anyway? *Paediatric and Perinatal Epidemiology 2*, 7–10.

Watt, A. (1986) Community health initiatives and their relation to general practice, *Journal of the Royal College of General Practitioners 36*, 72–3.

Whitehead, M. (1988) The Health Divide, in *Inequalities in Health*, Harmondsworth: Penguin.

Wilkinson, R. G. (ed.) (1986) *Class and Health: Research and Longitudinal Data*, London: Tavistock Publications.

World Health Organisation (1978) Declaration of Alma-Ata. *Lancet 2*, 1040–1.

World Health Organisation (1985) *Targets for Health For All*, Copenhagen: WHO Regional Office for Europe.

World Health Organisation, Health and Welfare Canada, Canadian Public Health Association (1986) *Ottawa Charter For Health Promotion* Copenhagen: WHO Regional Office for Europe.

World Health Organisation (1987a) *Health Promotion Concepts and Principles in Action – a Policy Framework*, Copenhagen: WHO Regional Office for Europe.

World Health Organisation (1987b) *Research Policy For Health For All*, Document EUR/RC37/5, Copenhagen: WHO Regional Office for Europe.

5

JULIAN LITTLE

CAN HEALTH BE PROMOTED?

The conceptual definition of health promotion is the '. . . process of enabling people to increase control over, and to improve, their health' (World Health Organisation, 1985). The key elements are recognition of the importance of behavioural issues in both prevention of specific disease and in the promotion of positive health, and the recognition that behavioural change cannot occur without reference to the 'total' environment: economic, physical, social and cultural.

What 'health promotion' is currently available in this country and to what extent do people take it up? This is a difficult question to answer as the conceptual definition is a basis which can give rise to an almost limitless number of issues. Five general subjects have been identified by the European region of the WHO and elaborated into 38 targets.

Access to health. Access to health covers reducing inequalities in health and increasing opportunities to improve health. The government did not implement the recommendations of the Black Report; it has been re-elected twice, and the final publication of the HEC *The Health Divide* (Whitehead, 1987) implies that inequalities have been widening. Paradoxically, however, the first of those 38 targets for health for all in Europe, all of which have been endorsed by the government of this country (Smith, 1986), is to reduce inequalities in health by 25 per cent by the year 2000.

Development of an environment conducive to health. Issues such as nuclear plants and acid rain generate a lot of attention in the

45

media but there is less enthusiasm for measures which require action by substantial proportions of the population, for example, for lead-free petrol or for cars equipped with exhaust catalysts.

Strengthening of social networks and social supports. The government sees community care of the elderly and mentally ill as a way of resolving the impossibility of extending state provision indefinitely (Fowler, 1986). Also, there are many self-help mutual-aid organisations but it's hard to keep track of increases and decreases in their activities (Gann, 1986).

Apart from this evidence of response to disease and infirmities as they arise there seems to be little evidence of strengthening of social networks and supports. The General Household Survey (1981) indicates that public involvement in action groups, be they tenants' associations or self-help groups, is a minority activity.

Promoting positive health behaviour. Most of the activity in this area has been formal health education, media coverage and books on healthy living. The results have been that most people are aware of the risks of smoking, excessive alcohol consumption, 'unsafe sex', a sedentary lifestyle and a poor diet and are aware to some extent of the benefits of screening. These issues are related to avoidance of negative health behaviour more than participation in positive health behaviour. Formal health education has, in fact, been the operational definition of health promotion. Experience with smoking, the most intensively studied health-related behaviour, suggests that rates of behaviour change are relatively slow and vary between different groups. In the case of smoking, the manual classes lag behind the non-manual classes. The evidence of the Black Report is that the groups in greatest need make least use of the preventive services (Townsend and Davidson, 1982).

Increasing knowledge and disseminating information about health. Again formal health education and media coverage have been important. The Health and Lifestyle survey has shown that the messages of health education about the behavioural cause of much disease have reached the younger groups in the population (Blaxter, 1987).

To sum up, when the operational definition of health promotion is followed – health education in avoidance of disease by way of behaviour change – then there is a lack of demand for health promotion. When the conceptual definition is followed, a lack of supply is apparent which is linked to the problems of welfare provision in general.

Especially in view of recent discussions about voucher systems (Klein, 1987), I want now to draw attention to one theory of the supply and demand of one aspect of welfare provision, notably the health services, which has some implication for the implementation of health promotion policies. This is the Theory of Public Choice advanced by Buchanan and Tollison (1972). The aim of their analysis was to link private choice, that is the behaviour of the buyer and seller in a fully competitive market, with public choice, typified by voting in purely democratic referenda in a single decision structure. The problem of the NHS, then, is that individuals engage in private choice behaviour as demanders of services and public choice of behaviour as voters and tax payers, who make decisions on supplying some of these services. The individual demands more services privately than he will supply publicly. The rational person would extend his demand on services to the point at which the overall perceived increase in benefit to him becomes zero. If he decides to reduce his demands on the grounds of social conscience, he is acting irrationally in that he is foregoing opportunities for personal gains without benefiting others to any measurable extent. When it comes to deciding about the supply of services the individual must balance costs against benefits. He must estimate the tax costs that various levels of service impose on him and weigh these against estimates of the benefits to be gained. It would be irrational for the individual to extend supply to the point where the increase in overall benefit to him from the services became zero because the sacrifice of alternatives would be relatively enormous. The individual's choice then, in the public choice context, will be for a quantity of investment in services much lower than that which would be required by a policy of providing services to the extent indicated by privately expressed 'needs'.

The novelty in this analysis lay in its extension of economic reasoning to political decisions. Its attraction as a theory lies in its simplicity. All that has to be acknowledged is that individual preferences are influential in determining political outcomes irrespective of the mechanism by which this process operates.

If this explanation is accepted, what are the implications for health promotion? First, the status quo: as already discussed, health services are in the condition of under-supply and over-demand (Table 5.1). Next, although it is difficult to generalise, pursuit of positive health behaviour is largely a private choice and

Table 5.1. Possible consequences of 'private' and 'public' choices about control of supply and demand on service provision

		CONTROL OF SUPPLY	
		PRIVATE CHOICE	PUBLIC CHOICE
	PRIVATE CHOICE	Market solution	Under-supply & over-demand
CONTROL OF DEMAND			
	PUBLIC CHOICE	Overall quality of services inadequate	Would eliminate congestion, stop deterioration in service standards, but would not resolve demand above limits 'chosen publicly'

so also is the supply of the facilities which enable the pursuit: food, leisure facilities and so on. As with all market solutions distributive results, in other words inequalities, follow. What can be done? We can reject the solution of making the control of demand a public choice and the control of supply a private choice, that is financing by voluntary contributions. This leaves, as a solution, a collective decision on how much services will be provided and how much services each member of society will have available to him. This would mean that there must be some clear allocation of services, either in terms of physical quantity units, for example, x visits to the surgery, y visits to the leisure centre, or in terms of more flexible units of general purchasing power. In theory, this would limit the growth of expenditure on the NHS and permit more resources to be directed into health promotion policies. How can such a shift in institutional structure be accomplished?

Some kind of social innovation is required. Rogers (1983) identifies four elements in the analysis of the diffusion of innovations:

(i) the innovation itself
(ii) communication of its existence
(iii) the social system, that in which the innovation occurs and in which it is diffused
(iv) the time dimension from innovation to its adoption (or rejection)

Stimulated by the experiences of North Karelia and perhaps some initiatives in Third World countries, some workers have suggested that health promotion initiatives will arise spontaneously in the community. It should be pointed out that North Karelia may not, in fact, be an example of spontaneous innovation. It has been pointed out that someone analysed heart disease figures and focused on North Karelia. However, in both the welfare and medical care areas, innovation has not been stimulated by public demand as such, it has been stimulated by needs as seen by the innovators. For example, in the 1950s sufferers from arthritis did not demand the replacement hip. This was developed by medical scientists and engineers on their own initiatives (Office of Health Economics, 1979). In the 1970s the Community Development Project was not a spontaneous demand of 12 deprived areas, it was the brainchild of a Civil Servant (Derek Morrell) working in the Home Office (Higgins *et al.*, 1983). Crofton (1987) has noted that, in Scotland, communities, when asked, did not spontaneously identify health problems. They focused first on other issues and then the workers assigned to the project tried to add to this a health Initiative. Moyan (Ginnety, 1987) and perhaps North Karelia seem exceptions rather than the rule. Thus, demand is effectively supplier-induced.

How can an innovation in the arena of health promotion become an option on which a public choice can be made? Diffusion research suggests that mass media channels are more effective in creating knowledge of innovations whereas interpersonal channels are more effective in informing and changing attitudes towards a new idea and thus influencing a decision to adopt or reject it. As regards health, the mass media channels would include the media itself, health education and pressure groups.

Over half the population belong to groups which at some time or other try to influence government policy, notably the trade unions (Jones and Kavanagh, 1979). Trade unions have sought to influence public and government thinking on a whole range of social and economic issues. Welfare issues have also been brought to public attention by the activities of sectional groups which defend and promote the interest of specific social groups, for example, Age

Concern, Shelter, and the Child Poverty Action Group. However, in the specific area of health, self-help groups have seldom been concerned with social change whereas they have blossomed in the areas of care (Calnan, 1986). Other health initiatives, for example scanner appeals, have provided for the acute services.

The general tendency for people to be interested in health questions only when they are ill themselves and then only in their own specific problem makes it difficult to generate a lot of interest in health at the local or neighbourhood level (Hatch, 1984). The new Public Health Alliance is to include voluntary groups. Should the emphasis be placed on sectional groups concerned with particular social issues and should trade unions also be involved? Such collaboration with other social movements would not be unlike that of two nineteenth-century movements with a profound influence on public health, the Phrenological Movement in Britain and the Popular Health Movement in America. Both were morally based, evangelical movements which were aligned with other radical social movements, especially those concerned with female emancipation (Williamson and Danaher, 1978).

As already mentioned, interpersonal channels of communication are more effective than the mass media channels in the process of deciding whether to adopt or reject an innovation. The results of an individual, A, telling B about the innovation are, to a large extent, determined by the social relationships of A and B. Rogers (1983) identified as one of the most important problems in the communication of innovations the fact that the participants are usually unlike one another in terms of belief, education, social status and so on. In theory at least, one way to resolve this problem is to decentralise the diffusion system. Thus, health would be promoted through community initiatives. This approach has the obvious merits of (1) being small-scale and (2) the possibility that vested interests are less likely to be influential than is the case for national initiatives.

In this country collective action at neighbourhood level directed towards health questions is a recent phenomenon (Hatch, 1984). Some such actions have followed the community development model, that is, one in which change is achieved through consensus. Community development is client-centred and based on the self-determined goals of the community groups with which the worker is involved (Bryant, 1972). The Health Education Council funded a number of community development experiments in the 5 years before it was disbanded (Whitehead, 1987). For example, in an inner-city area in Catford, the feasibility of a community health council employing a health worker to help local people identify and act on their health needs was explored (Reason, 1985). Most of the other projects have also arisen in the context of attempts to respond to the problems of inner-city areas: for example, the housing project in Edinburgh (Martin *et al.*, 1987) and the Waterloo project in London (Miller, 1980). So far as I am aware, there has been little evaluation of these initiatives as yet. However, a number of problems have been identified in the course of other community development projects.

First, the notion of community has proved to be a romantic ideal. Social loyalties in what are commonly described as communities are diverse and complex (Jones *et al.*, 1983). These loyalties vary according to the issue considered. Studies in North America have shown that different small groups make decisions on different community problems (Polsby, 1969). Therefore, consensus on a health promotion package, which will involve decisions affecting many different aspects of community life, is unlikely. In the poverty programmes of the Kennedy era in the United States, local groups did not work through conflict to reach consensus (Jones *et al.*, 1983).

Second, the majority are not interested in participation. In a survey carried out on behalf of the Commission on the Constitution in the early 1970s only a low level of interest in political and community affairs was found (Klein, 1984). Moreover, those most heavily involved tended to be from the most advantaged groups. Forty-four per cent of professionals and managers were rated as being 'very involved' as compared to only 10 per cent of unskilled workers and 21 per cent of skilled workers.

Third, the leaders who do emerge are often no more representative than local government officials. The public forums which emerged in response to the Skeffington Report, in which greater public participation in physical planning was advocated, proved to be either exercises in manipulation by town-hall staff or monopolised by small but strident pressure groups (Jones *et al.*, 1983).

If an attempt is made to target a group suffering the worse health, then, as Watt (1986) has pointed out, despite the similarity of background, social relationships may not be harmonious.

Community action is a parallel process to community development but uses conflict to achieve change (Bryant, 1972). As a strategy it is open to the same limitations as community development but, in practice, goals tend to be narrower so there tend to be fewer tensions between different local interest groups. Experience in the social welfare area indicates that the major factor determining the effectiveness of the action is the nature of the issue which is the focus for action. Issues which require modification of local administrative procedures and practices, for example dust bin collections, are more likely to be won than those which require major policy and political changes.

One example is particularly pertinent as regards health promotion. The Community Development Project was set up in 1969 by the Home Office in collaboration with local authorities in deprived neighbourhoods of different kinds. The original aims were:
(1) To study the needs of the areas.
(2) To help public services working in them formulate more effective and more closely co-ordinated programmes to meet these needs.
(3) To focus public attention, locally and nationally, on these needs.
(4) To give people in the areas a voice in the debate and opportunities for doing things themselves (Donnison, 1980).

These aims correspond in no small degree with the WHO's general subjects for health promotion in Europe. However, the project leaders were not content with local, small-scale amelioration and changed the aim to educating local people about what they, the project leaders, saw as the fundamental causes of inequalities in the political and economic system so that local people could create pressure for change (Donnison, 1980). In the end, the Community Development Project teams argued that there were building links from the bottom of the political system within groups that represented the working class. In the concluding stages of the project the team sought funding in turn from the Home Office, the Social Science Research Council, the Gulbenkian, Rowntree, Nuffield, Cadbury and Sainsbury Foundations but there was to be no 'subsidised revolution'. The government quietly terminated the project in 1977. Brynmor John, announcing termination of the project in the House of Commons, claimed that it had had a 'negative result' and that it had principally taught the government 'what not to do' (Hansard, 17th November: cited by Higgins *et al.*, 1983). The basic limitation of the approach, therefore, is that bodies with resources to effect major economic and political changes are unlikely to sponsor projects which threaten dissent against themselves.

In conclusion, it is no surprise that there has been so little progress in health promotion according to the conceptual definition. According to the Theory of Public Choice, individual decisions about providing health services and the infrastructure for health promotion are matters of public choice, whereas use of health services and health promoting behaviours are matters of private choice. If this is accepted as an explanation, one way for progress to be achieved is to remove this inconsistency in decision making. Such an innovation is unlikely to arise spontaneously, and the suggested method by which it might eventually be adopted is through sectional groups concerned with particular social issues and trades unions.

Previous experience in the area of welfare provision suggest that what can be achieved from community-based initiatives is limited. The aims of such initiatives should be modest and the initiatives themselves should be based on existing groups. Participation might be expected to raise awareness of the broader policy issues involved but not to lead directly to changes in policy. Ultimately, however, we would hope for a recognition that, in David Hume's words: 'Public utility is the sole origin of justice'.

References

Blaxter, M. (1987). Beliefs about the causes of health and ill–health, in B. D. Cox et al., The Health and Lifestyle Survey, pp.131–40, London: Health Promotion Research Trust.

Bryant, R. (1972). Community action, Br. J. Social Work, 2: 205–15.

Buchanan, J. M. and Tollison, R. D. (1972). Theory of Public Choice: Political Application of Economics, Ann Arbor: University of Michigan Press.

Calnan (1986) in S. Rodmell and A. Watt (eds), The Politics of Health Education : Raising the Issues, London : Routledge & Kegan Paul.

Donnison, D. (1980). Urban development and social policies, in R. A. B. Leaper (ed.), Health, Wealth and Housing, Oxford: Blackwell & Robertson.

Fowler, N. (1986). Speech to the Association of Directors of Social Services, Cardiff, September 1986, cited in New Society, 18th September, p.1 of supplement.

Gann, R. (1986). The Health Information Handbook, Aldershot: Gower.

General Household Survey 1977 (1981). Social Trends, 11: 186.

Hatch, S. (1984). Participation in health, in R. Maxwell and N. Weaver (eds.), Public Participation in Health: Towards a Clearer View, p.101–12. London: King's Fund.

Higgins, J., Deakin, N., Edwards, J., and Wicks, M. (1983). *Government and Urban Poverty*, Oxford: Blackwell.

Jones, B. and Kavanagh, D. (1979). *British Politics Today : A Student's Guide*, Manchester: Manchester University Press.

Jones, K., Brown, J. and Bradshaw, J. (1983). *Issues in Social Policy*, London: Routledge & Kegan Paul.

Klein, R. (1984). The politics of participation, in R. Maxwell and N. Weaver (eds), *Public Participation in Health: Towards a Clearer View*, p. 17–32. London: King's Fund.

Klein, R. (1987). The case for a voucher system, *New Society* supplement on 'Care in the Community', 18th September 1987, p.12.

Martin, C. J., Hunt, S. M. and Platt, S. D. (1987). Illness experience in a community: whose responsibility? Society for Social Medicine, 31st Annual Scientific Meeting, Dublin, 16th–18th September 1987.

Miller, J. (1980) The Waterloo health project, in J. Hudley (ed.), *Community Work and Health*, Paisley College of Technology Local Government Unit.

Office of Health Economics (1979) Scarce Resources in Health Care London, OHE.

Polsby, N. W. (1968) Study of community power, in Sills, D. L. (ed.), *International Encylopaedia of the Social Sciences*, Vol.3, p.157, London: Crown Collier & Macmillan; New York: Free Press.

Reason, L. (1985) *Catford Community Health Project: Evaluation Report*, Report to Health Education Council.

Rogers, E. M. (1983) *Diffusion of Innovations* (3rd edn), New York: Free Press.

Royal Commission on the Constitution (1973) Devaluation and other aspects of government: an attitudes survey. Research paper no.7, London: HMSO.

Smith, R. (1986) Whatever happened to the Black report? *Br. Med. J.*, *293*, 91–2.

Townsend, P. and Davidson, N. (eds) (1982) *Inequalities in Health: The Black Report*, Harmondsworth: Penguin.

Watt, A. (1986) Community health education: a time for caution? in S. Rodmeu and A. Watt (eds), *The Politics of Health Education: Raising the Issues*, pp.139–64, London: Routledge and Kegan Paul.

Whitehead, M. (1987) *The Health Divide: Inequalities in Health in the 1980s*, London: Health Education Council.

Williamson, J. D. and Danaher, K. (1978) *Self-care in Health*, London: Croom-Helm.

World Health Organisation Regional Office for Europe (1985) *Targets for Health for All*, Copenhagen: WHO.

Inequalities in Health

6

SALLY MACINTYRE, ELLEN ANNANDALE, RUSSELL ECOB,
GRAEME FORD, KATE HUNT, BARBARA JAMIESON,
SHEILA MACIVER, PATRICK WEST, AND SALLY WYKE

THE WEST OF SCOTLAND TWENTY-07 STUDY:
HEALTH IN THE COMMUNITY

The West of Scotland Twenty–07 Study: Health in the Community involves prospective surveys of everyday life and health among three age cohorts (15-, 35- and 55-year-olds) resident within a large and relatively heterogeneous region in the Glasgow area. It is intended to follow the three cohorts prospectively over a 20-year period, collecting data about individuals and the social and physical milieux they inhabit. Data are being collected to compare life circumstances, beliefs, behaviours and health within and between ages, over time and between areas which will allow us to develop and test models of the relationship between social position and health.

Design features intended to facilitate the linking of these different types of data include (a) a regional sample consisting of 52 post-code sectors on a continuum of social deprivation and (b) the selection of two localities in Glasgow for intensive focus, studying features which might promote or inhibit health or the opportunity to live healthy lives.

The first wave of data collection is still under way. In the absence of results, we wish to highlight some of the research issues which provide the rationale for the study and to outline the main features of the research design. We begin by describing the general background of the study and then draw out some of the issues specific to the three age cohorts.

The study rationale
The study aims to integrate an older tradition of examining material

56

and environmental influences on the health of the population with the more recent emphasis on the importance of personal behaviours and psychosocial factors. It also aims to study the relative importance of health selection and social causation explanations for social differentials in health, and, most importantly, it provides the opportunity to study the mechanisms by which such processes – selection and social causation – might work.

It is important to stress that while some commentators (cf. Black, 1980; Doyal *et al.*, 1983) have treated structuralist/materialist/environmental' and 'cultural/behavioural/lifestyle' factors as contrasting explanations for the social patterning of health, we do not see them as necessarily mutually exclusive. Similarly, we do not assume that health selection or social causation explanations for social inequalities in health have to be mutually exclusive. Rather, we think that it is important to try to determine *the balance* between these types of explanations under particular sets of conditions, and to explore in empirical detail exactly how they operate. Thus we are addressing the questions: under what conditions does selection by health occur, and by what mechanisms?; within a social causation model, what is the relative importance of material and psycho-social factors, voluntary and constrained factors?; and under what sorts of circumstances and by which mechanisms do they operate?

It is important to note also that we are not assuming that health selection constitutes a form of social Darwinism or is simply consequential on genetic or biological factors. While characteristics such as sex and age are biologically based, their classification is importantly shaped by culture (Finch, 1986; Morgan, 1986). Thus, the processes involved in selection by health may be profoundly social, and only understandable in the light of the specific cultural contexts in which individuals conduct their everyday lives.

Much of the empirical and conceptual background to the *West of Scotland Twenty-07 Study* has been published elsewhere (Macintyre, 1986a). That review paper documents the extensive empirical evidence of the associations between health (variously measured) and six social positions – social (occupational) class, gender, marital status, age, ethnicity and area of residence. The argument developed from the discussion about the causal processes underlying these associations, is that we need more prospective sociological research on unselected populations to explore, empirically, the processes linking social position and health.

Before describing the study in more detail, it is pertinent briefly

Figure 6.1. Mortality of men and women in different regions of Britain, 1979–80 plus 1982–83

Region	Direct age-standardised death rate (per 1,000)		
	Men 20–64	Single women 20–59	Married women 20–59
Central Clydeside	7.86	1.78	3.23
Strathclyde	7.14	1.66	3.06
North	6.43	1.56	2.50
North West	6.37	1.69	2.52
Remainder of Scotland	6.13	1.47	2.58
Wales	5.86	1.43	2.34
Yorks and Humberside	5.83	1.48	2.32
West Midlands	5.72	1.54	2.26
East Midlands	5.28	1.40	2.14
South East	4.88	1.29	1.97
South West	4.82	1.32	1.93
East Anglia	4.37	1.14	1.79
Scotland	6.92	1.62	2.89
England and Wales	5.43	1.41	2.17
Britain	5.57	1.43	2.23

Source: Whitehead (1987), p.25.

to locate it in three broad contexts – historical, geographical and conceptual.

The historical context. The study is being conducted during a time of quite intense debate about social class inequalities in health; relating for example, to problems of measurement, the extent to which inequalities are widening or narrowing and whether they are the outcome of processes of selection or social causation (Fox, Goldblatt and Jones, 1985; Hart, 1986; Illsley, 1986; Townsend and Davidson, 1982; Wilkinson, 1986).

There were increasing differentials in specific-cause death rates between manual and non-manual classes over the years 1970–72 and 1979–83 in Britain (Marmot and McDowell, 1986). We point to these data to underscore the continuing importance of health inequalities, the validity and interpretation of which has been hotly debated. This is understandable since they have fundamental significance for both social theories, and for health and welfare policies. However, the type and level of data needed to address many of the issues is often unavailable. For example, the only empirical evidence often quoted in relation to selection theories is Illsley's (1955) work on the relationship between height, social mobility of *women* at marriage and their subsequent perinatal outcomes. As much of the work is cross-sectional (e.g. the Decennial Supplements), it has not been possible to separate out cause and effect and explore the relative importance of social causation and social selection. Other work in this area (e.g. the Longitudinal Study; Fox and Goldblatt, (1982)) is restricted to data derived from routinely gathered statistics. Although our study does not solely focus on class inequalities, it was influenced by the social class debate and the type of research design (for example, prospective) and data (wide-ranging measures of everyday life and of health) that is necessary to resolve some of these complex questions.

The geographical context. The West of Scotland has a generally poor health record compared with the rest of Scotland, the UK, and other developed countries. Whitehead (1987) shows that, for men and women seperately, the Central Clydeside Conurbation had the highest age-standardised death rates of all regions in Britain (Figure 1). However, within the West of Scotland there is considerable variation in health (at least as measured by death rates).

A more detailed picture of mortality in the Greater Glasgow Health Board area (GGHB, 1986) shows that, in the early 1980s, the areas having the highest mortality had mortality ratios which were two and a half times those of the areas with the lowest mortality. For some causes of death there was an even greater difference – for example, for lung cancer a five-fold difference is observed. In the areas with lowest mortality, death rates were as low as those in the healthiest countries of the world, such as Sweden or Japan. Thus, in spite of its overall poor record, the West of Scotland has such a spread of health experience that it is an ideal location for studying how the social and physical environment might influence health.

The conceptual focus. The Twenty–07 Study is attempting to explore and explain observed associations between social position and a broad range of health outcomes, rather than trying to explain the social aetiology of specific diseases. We are thus interested in taking an extensive view of health along a number of different dimensions (mental and physical health, vulnerability to ill health, functional capacity, fitness, the cumulative impact of disease, etc.) and looking at the processes linking these with the occupancy of various social positions. This is not to imply that

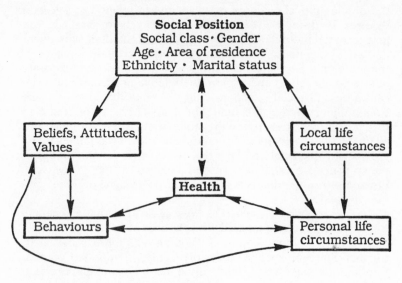

Figure 6.2.

the social positions in question *necessarily* involve generalised vulnerability to, or protection from, ill health, but to suggest that unless a range of health outcomes is examined, it is not possible to address the question of the specificity or generality of health risks by reference to these social positions. As well as taking a broadly based view of health, we are trying to take as extensive a view as we can of possible influences on health. The study therefore involves a wide-ranging and large data-collection exercise.

Figure 2 shows the general model underlying the study. It starts with the observed relationship between the six *social positions* and health (variously measured). Figure 2 acknowledges the fact that health has social consequences (for example, employability, educability, social mobility, dependence, family functioning, etc.) as well as social causes. We hypothesise that four broad groups of variables – personal life circumstances; local life circumstances, beliefs, attitudes and values; and behaviours – are related to social position and shaped by the wider social structure and historical context. The relationship of each of these groups of variables with each of the others, and with health, may be in either direction; behaviour can create life circumstances or life circumstances constrain behaviours; beliefs, attitudes or values may either shape, or

Figure 6.3.

Health

Self-assessed – General health, vulnerability fitness, physique, vision, hearing

Self-reported – Illness, chronic conditions, dental condition, medical/surgical history, mental health, disability, malaise

Directly measured – Height, weight, blood pressure, respiratory function, girth, reaction times

Behaviours

Use of time
Paid and unpaid work
Exercise at work, home and leisure
Diet
Alcohol use
Smoking
Recreational activities
Sex
Contraception
Sleep
Contacts with friends/kin
Illness behaviour
Use of Health Services
Medication
Religious activities
Preventive health behaviour

Beliefs, attitudes and values

Concepts of health
Beliefs about causes of health and ill health
Health knowledge (re smoking, alcohol use, diet, etc.)
Religious beliefs
Personal concerns (worries about various life domains)
Beliefs about age, sex and marital appropriate roles
Satisfaction with various life domains
Opinion scales
Self esteem
Coping strategies

Life circumstances – personal

Biography
Family formation
Household and family composition
Illness in family members
Type and quality of accommodation
Housing tenure
Amenities (cars, telephone, garden, household amenities)
Occupation
Economic activity
Place and type of work (paid or unpaid)
Income, wealth, benefits
Domestic division of labour and family responsibilities
Migration
Kinship networks

Life circumstances – local

Housing stock and policies
Transport and traffic
Land use
Educational and training facilities
Recreational facilities
Crime and policing
Community activities and participation
Food and other retail outlets
Environmental hazards (noise, airborne pollution, etc.)
Primary health care
Secondary health care
Welfare services
Employment opportunities and labour market

be shaped by, behaviours, etc. Life circumstances, beliefs or behaviours can all be hypothesised to influence health either directly or via the mechanism of one or two of the others. Figure 3 lists some of the areas which will be explored under each heading.

Where we differ from the voluntaristic lifestyle models which focus on beliefs, attitudes and values (the left hand side of Figure 2) is in taking life circumstances (both personal and local) much more seriously than has often been the case.

The study design

Details of the study population and sampling frame are described in Ecob (1987) and are only outlined in brief here. As noted above, the sample comprises a 'regional' sample and two 'locality' samples; the former is a two-stage, stratified random sample, comprising 52 post-code sectors (clusters) randomly selected from the Central Clydeside conurbation with probability proportional to their total population.

The regional sample was selected in the following way. The 203 post-code sectors in the Central Clydeside Conurbation were stratified first by area (combining the local government districts into six strata) and, then within area by two social indicators chosen on the basis of their correlation with all-cause mortality. These were the proportion of individuals over 16 not in employment, and the proportion of economically active in low-earning socio-economic groups; their correlations with all-cause mortality at around the 1981 census were the highest of all the census variables considered, and were 0.84 and 0.85 respectively. The sampling fraction in our 52 post-code sectors is lower than in our localities. On average, around 20 per cent of those in the particular age groups in each cluster were selected. The target sample size across these small areas is 1,000 per cohort.

The localities selected for intensive investigation are in the North West and South West of the city of Glasgow, with populations at the 1981 census of 50 and 60 thousand respectively. In 1980–82, the all-cause standardised mortality ratios for those aged 0–64 were 83 in the North West and 114 in the South West. The North West is a more middle class, and the South West a more working class area, though neither are at the extremes of social class composition (MacIver, 1988). Within these localities we are surveying virtually the entire population of 15-, 35- and 55-year-olds – around 300 per cohort per locality.

The regional and locality samples provide the two main vehicles for studying what we have called 'local life circumstances' (see

Figure 2). The first involves an analysis of area effects which derive from the fact that each cluster can be located along a continuum from the most to the least socially deprived. The second is a much more comprehensive study of the two localities focusing on both their social and physical properties. Thus, we are collecting data on a wide range of factors such as the health and welfare services, recreational facilities, employment opportunities, housing, transport and retail food outlets. These data will enable us to study the ways in which these factors might inhibit or promote their residents' health and opportunities to lead healthy lives.

The same interview schedules are being administered to members of the locality and regional samples. The regional sample (within which the two selected smaller localities are situated) provides us with expected population values so that the statistical comparisons can be made between areas. Area-based data can be combined with information collected on individuals which will allow us to work systematically back and forth between individuals and their social and physical milieux. We will then be able to test models of the social production of health and the relative importance of the personal or environmental, or material and psychosocial, influences on health. Hypotheses on possible area influences on health derived from the more qualitative comparison of the two localities can be tested on the larger regional sample.

In the first sweep of data collection respondents are interviewed in their own homes by a trained interviewer. In the case of 15-year-olds, there is also a separate interview with parents conducted by another interviewer on the same occasion to obtain information on the family's history and circumstances. Respondents are subsequently visited by a nurse who asks more detailed questions on health, and measures height, weight, blood pressure, respiratory function and reaction times (Macintyre, 1986b). Sample members also complete a few short questionnaires in their own time and give them to the nurse when he or she calls. The intention is to reinterview sample members at approximately 5-yearly intervals, and in some circumstances to recontact respondents for a telephone interview or postal questionnaire at shorter intervals. The fieldwork for the 15- and 35-year-old cohorts is nearly complete, and that for the 55-year-olds is under way.

The age cohorts

Having outlined the general background to and features of the study design, we now go on to focus more specifically on the age-cohort component of the Twenty–07 Study. Age is, of course, a significant variable for research on health-related outcomes. However, its treatment in social research has often been problematic. Often quite broad age groupings are used (to avoid the problem of small cell numbers). When such broad groupings (for example, the OPCS classification of 0–15, 16–44, 45–64 and 65 plus) are used it becomes difficult, if not impossible, to appreciate the medical and social significance of such states as 'unemployment', 'parenthood', 'divorce' and the interrelationships between them. By holding age constant and taking three single-year cohorts, we will have a more economical sample size and will be able to explore variation in physiological and 'social' age around the same chronological age and to consider differences between age groups with greater confidence.

The three age cohorts (15-, 35- and 55-year-olds) have been chosen to represent slices of the life course. Although most of the topics and measures used in the study are applied across the three age groups, there are obviously many age specific concerns in addition to these.

The 15-year-old cohort. By comparison with the two older cohorts, 15-year-olds share certain common characteristics which are a direct function of their age: they are still (officially) at school, typically reside in the parental home, are not yet entitled to marry, and in a variety of other ways, are designated as 'minors' by reference to legal and social norms (West, 1986). Within a relatively short period of time, however, this *relative* uniformity in social position is transformed into a remarkable diversity of positions, statuses and life experiences. The collection of baseline health data, therefore, provides a major opportunity to study both the effect of health on social position and the effect of social position on health over a period of critical change that characterises the transition from youth to adulthood.

To illustrate the potential that this cohort affords to understanding the relative importance of these processes and the mechanisms by which they occur, we will focus our attention in this paper on the issue of class differentials. Of all the ways health varies by social parameters, social class continues to attract most attention, in large part, of course, because of the controversy about the explanation of class inequalities. The 15-year-old cohort is ideally suited to explore the relative importance of health selection and social causation, and the processes involved, as young people move from their social class of origin to their achieved social class within a period of approximately 10 years.

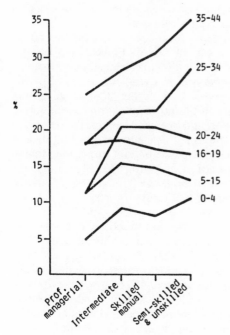

Figure 6.4. Chronic illness (%) by social class (HOH) in childhood, youth and early adulthood.
Source: Secondary Analysis of General Household Survey, 1980.

This focus on what happens between youth and adulthood in terms of class position achieves greater significance when it is appreciated that, on available evidence, the situation in youth is characterised more by the absence than the presence of class differentials in health, but that the familiar pattern of inequalities emerges (or re-emerges) fairly soon in early adulthood (Lundberg, 1986; West, in press). If this is surprising, it is only because, in the more accessible published data on this issue, the pattern in youth, and indeed at other specific stages in the life course, is entirely obscured by the very broad age bands employed. The picture is illustrated in Figure 4 using data derived from the 1980 General Household Survey (Gilbert *et al.*, 1983).

The gradients refer to rates of 'chronic illness' defined as the percentage reporting 'longstanding illness, disability or infirmity' or, in those aged under 16, an equivalent report by an adult. Social class is based on the occupation of the head of household (HoH): in the under–16-year-olds, this is usually a parent and, over that age, it refers either to the individual's own occupation or, in the case of married women, to the husband's occupation.

Figure 4 shows that in the first few years of life (0–4) a social class gradient is apparent. At 5–15 years, except for an increase between the professional/managerial and intermediate social classes, there is no evidence of a gradient. At 16–19 years the pattern is almost reversed, and in the 20–24 age group, again excepting the low rate in the professional/managerial class. no gradient is observed. By 25 and in ensuing years, the pattern of class differentials is (re-)established as a steeper gradient than in the youngest age group. Using own occupation, rather than that of HoH, results in a similar pattern in youth (16–19) though the re-emerging gradient occurs earlier at age 20–24. The picture for males and females is very similar.

This pattern of relative equalisation in youth, and the re-establishment of class gradients in early adulthood, is observable in respect of other indicators of health such as mortality and self-rated health (West, in press). Furthermore, a similar widening of class differentials in respect to health-related behaviours like smoking and alcohol consumption appears to characterise the period between youth and adulthood. On available evidence, rather more similarity than difference between social classes in youth is observed (Fogelman, 1976; Plant *et al.*, 1985; Gillies, 1987). The question posed by these data is, how does the youth pattern get transformed into the much more familiar adult pattern within such a relatively short time span?

One possible explanation for the change in pattern between youth and early adulthood is *health selection*; healthier youngsters experience upward social mobility, less healthy ones downward mobility. That this might be at least part of the answer is suggested by the fact that it is in youth, or more precisely at entry into the labour market, that perhaps the major process of sorting or allocation of individuals into occupational roles occurs. Our interest here is not simply confined to a comparison of the before/after type but involves a focus on the processes involved, both by reference to the trajectories or routes followed after the end of statutory education and the mechanisms by which selection actually occurs.

In respect of trajectories, we will be in a position to see how health as an independent variable (measured at age 15) affects the likelihood of remaining in further education, entering the Youth Training Scheme (YTS), becoming unemployed and so on. In very general terms, we would hypothesise that the complexity of the current situation compared with the once simple school-to-work transition (Carter, 1962; Veness 1962) could mean that the impact of health selection is considerable. In a highly competitive market with an ever increasing number of agencies controlling entry into, and movement within, the labour market, health as a resource is likely to matter more for occupational achievement than ever before.

In respect of the mechanisms by which health selection occurs, what we refer to are the characteristics or attributes of individuals which underpin such selection. Here, a distinction can be made between *direct* and *indirect* mechanisms. The first constitutes health selection in its overt or explicit form (i.e. 'health' itself directly affects opportunities in the labour market). The second involves all those other attributes which affect opportunities in the labour market, the most important of which, of course, is ability or educational achievement. In addition, we are also focusing on the possible effects of differences in social identity, principally expressed in terms of conventional and unconventional youth styles, and physical attractiveness which has received almost no attention outside the rather narrow confines of experimental psychology. Each of these, to a greater or lesser extent, may influence an individual's occupational career and hence achieved social class position. Inasmuch as each is associated with health, the net (implicit) effect of such occupational mobility is health selection.

Health selection, of course is not the only (nor even the most likely) explanation of the (re-)emergence of class differentials in early childhood. An alternative stresses either the notion of a time delay in the effects of early environment and/or the (compounding) influence of factors such as the working environment or behaviours like smoking later in life. In order to demonstrate the importance of such social factors for health, however, it is essential that we take account of the role of health selection. Its potential significance is not confined to social class but extends as one possible explanation of the association between employment status or marital status and health. Are those who become unemployed already less healthy? Are those who get married more healthy in advance of their marriage? In short, to what extent are the associations between social positions and health observed at later ages a consequence of earlier health selection processes.

The 35-year-old cohort. In exploring the association between social position and health, the 35-year-old cohort provides an excellent opportunity to investigate the diversity of circumstances and experience that inhere within a group of individuals of the same chronological age. Both because of ageing and cohort effects, we expect to find a wide variety of experience across events and statuses (such as marital status, work status and family formation) thought to be associated with physical and mental health status.

Two areas which we see as central to the 35-year-old cohort are experiences in the family and in work. There is, of course, a large body of literature addressing the relationship between work, marital status and health, especially in their association with gender. For example, data on marital status and health have shown that death rates are higher for the non-married compared to the married (Fox and Goldblatt, 1982; Verbrugge, 1983). There is also some indication that the health protective effect of marriage may disproportionately benefit men (Gove, 1973). Much research, too, has pointed to the higher prevalence of morbidity (variously measured) amongst women compared to men (Nathanson, 1977; Gove and Hughes, 1979).

However, one problem associated with much research in this tradition has been the insensitive measurement of variables such as marital status, work experience and gender. We know little about what exactly it *is* about marriage or gender which produces differential experience of health, illness and death. The intention, therefore, is to move beyond the normative assumptions that are implicit in the measurement of statuses like 'being married', 'being single', 'male' and 'female', or 'in paid work'. Our analysis will not simply be confined to these categories, but will take into account the diversity of *experience* that lies within them. For example, in respect to marital status, the relationship between home and work life (using measures that are applicable to both unpaid domestic work in the home and paid employment), domestic work, the domestic division of labour, and patterns of reproduction will be explored. In considering gender and health we will be looking not only at the experience of being male or female but also general role ideology and dimensions of 'maleness' and 'femaleness' (Bem, 1981).

Born in 1951 or 1952 at the tail end of the 'baby boom' generation of the post-war period, this cohort were in their teens in the late 1960s and experienced (though obviously to varying degrees) the large-scale cultural and social changes that took place during this period. Two specific issues which deserve particular attention in this cohort are increasing educational opportunities

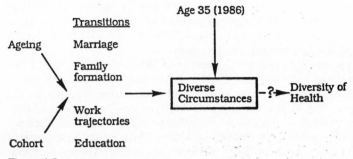

Figure 6.5.

(especially for women), and changes in patterns of marriage and family formation. Some 35-year-olds will be unmarried, others just entering marriage and/or starting a family, while still others will have teenage children, some of whom will have already left home. This cohort is also likely to experience a quite high level of marital dissolution and divorce. Related to this, we are likely to see a relatively high percentage of single parent families, especially single mothers.

Linked to the expected diversity in patterns of family formation, the cohort is significant in the context of changing legislation and provision of abortion and contraception. Abortion was legalised in 1967 immediately prior to our sample becoming sexually active, and the birth control pill only became widely available to single women in the early 1970s (*Lancet*, Editorial, 1985). Detailed reproductive and contraceptive histories have been collected from women and we are particularly interested in both the association of contraceptive practice and health, and its effect on health through its influence upon reproduction, marital status, family formation, and living arrangements.

One further historical issue that we think is important for this cohort is work. Many women in the sample will have grown up with the expectation of working outside the home and 35-year-old men, too, will have left school with expectations of full employment. Of particular interest will be the relatively high level of female involvement in the work force in association with unprecedented levels of male unemployment (Strathclyde Regional Council, 1987).

We will be focusing upon the way in which our sample have passed through several critical transitions (see Figure 5) such as education, marriage, family formation and work. Our principle analytic interest lies in exploring the associations between diversity

The West of Scotland Twenty-07 Study 70

in circumstances and diversity in health, giving special attention to the tensions and continuities that are part of everyday life as experience in family, work and leisure. We will also be examining patterns of stress and social support.

Having highlighted the diversity of circumstances at age 35, it is important to emphasise that we do not see the differential experience of the sample as lying solely, or even principally, in indivudal choice. As Figure 5 illustrates, we envisage the current circumstances of the sample to be mediated by the six social positions that form the core of the Twenty–07 Study. Thus, educational opportunities and entry into the labour force, age at marriage and reproductive patterns, to give a few examples, are likely to be significantly influenced by the cultural and material context in which our sample live and the constraints of social class position and gender.

We expect health differentials to be well established by age 35. Some indication of social class differentials and health, for example, can be seen in data from the General Household Survey presented in Figure 5. We will be looking at the six social structural variables and giving particular attention to their interaction with, and possibly independent effects of, family work and leisure patterns upon health.

The 55-year-old cohort. By comparison to other age groups, the middle-aged have been neglected in health-related studies. There is a large body of research on the social, economic and health problems faced by elderly people. Yet, surprisingly, the possibility that these problems might have their roots in circumstances and decisions made in late middle age has received little attention. The longitudinal design of the Twenty–07 Study offers the opportunity to examine the interactions between social and economic circumstances and individual experience of health and illness and their longer term impact on problems in old age.

Many 55-year-olds are beginning to experience serious ill health. Indeed, 22 per cent of 55-year-old men, and 12 per cent of women, are expected to die by the time they are 65 (Bosanquet, 1987). Most of this mortality is concentrated in certain social groups, for example, the Standardised Mortality Ratios (SMRs) of men aged 55–64 range from 55 for those in social class I, to 110 for those in social class IV. In respect of morbidity, data from the Third National Morbidity Study (Royal College of General Practitioners, 1986) show that while the number of 'trivial' and 'intermediate' episodes of illness presented to physicians was minimally high in the 45–64 year-olds compared to 25–44 year-olds, the number of *serious* episodes was two and a half times greater. Thus, by comparison with the two younger cohorts, we can expect to find a wide range of morbidity and health service use in the sample.

The 55-year-old cohort was born during the Depression of 1933 and experienced the austerity of war-time and post-war Britain during the early years of their lives. Most married, and went on to have children, in the 'boom years' of the 1950s and 1960s. Now, in the 1980s, many face early retirement or redundancy. The cumulative impact of these life-time experiences may have direct consequences for their health, health-related behaviours, and attitudes to life.

Full-time work up to retirement at the age of 65 used to be the norm, but will soon be the exception (Bosanquet, 1987). In 1985, 39 per cent of Scottish men were either economically inactive or unemployed. Unemployment at this age is likely to be long-term with individuals having little prospect of rejoining the labour force. Early retirement is also increasingly common, but whereas in the 1970s it was usually due to ill-health, in the 1980s it occurs for a much wider diversity of reasons, such as compulsory or voluntary redundancy. These changes in employment status will obviously be experienced differently according to how individuals are situated by reference to the social positions of interest.

Contrary to the usual view of late middle-age as a time of little change, we consider 55-year-olds to be entering a dynamic period of their lives. Some changes may be a direct consequence of either their own morbidity or the morbidity or mortality of significant others. Further, women may be experiencing the physiological, psychological, and social changes associated with the immediate post-menopausal years. Compounding the impact of health-related problems on the lives of 55-year-olds are changes in their family situation. They are a 'generation in the middle'. Their own children may have left home, but they may be directly involved in caring for grandchildren at the same time as their own parents become increasingly dependent.

While there are some well known community studies of health in the United States (Berkman and Breslow, 1983; Kessler and Levin, 1970; Koos, 1954), there have been few conducted in Britain and their full potential has rarely been realised. The West of Scotland Twenty–07 Study: Health in the Community is designed to provide more comprehensive explanations of well documented differentials in health. The age cohorts, selected to represent critical phases in the life-course, should, in the long term, enable an assessment to be made of the relative importance of health selection and social causation, not merely in respect of class inequalities, but of other less prominent, but no less important, differentials.

Within and between cohorts, it should also be possible to identify the balance between 'structuralist/materialist/environmental' and 'cultural/behavioural/lifestyle' factors in their impact upon health. Finally, because data are being systematically collected on the characteristics of the two localities, within which survey respondents are located, we are not just dependent on data collected at the level of individuals. The effect of local life circumstances, both physical and social, on the health of individuals can be determined.

References

Bem, S. L. (1981) *Bem Sex-Role Inventory Professional Manual*, Palo Alto, Calif: Consulting Psychologists Press.

Berkman, L. and Breslow, L. H. (1983) *Health and Ways of Living: The Alameda County Study*, Oxford: Oxford University Press.

Black, D. (1980) *Inequalities in Health: Report of a Working Group*, London: DHSS/HMSO.

Bosanquet, N. (1987) *A Generation in Limbo. Government, The Economy and the 55_65 Age Group in Britain*, London: Public Policy Centre.

Carter, M. (1962) *Home, School and Work*, Oxford: Pergamon.

Doyal, L., Green, K., Irwin, A., Russell, D., Stewart, F., Williams, R., Gee, D. and Epstein, S. (1983) *Cancer in Britain: The Politics of Prevention*, London: Pluto Press.

Ecob, R. (1987) *West of Scotland Twenty-07 Study: The Sampling Scheme, Frame and Procedures for the Cohort Studies*, MRC Medical Sociology Unit Working Paper No.6.

Finch, J. (1986) 'Age', in R. Burgess (ed.), *Key Variables in Social Investigation*, London: RKP.

Fogelman, K. (1976) *Britain's Sixteen Year Olds*, London: National Children's Bureau.

Fox, A. J. and Goldblatt, P. O. (1982) *Longitudinal Study: Sociodemographic mortality differentials*, London: OPCS, HMSO.

Fox, A. J., Goldblatt, P. O. and Jones, D. R. (1985) Social class mortality differences: artefact, selection or life circumstances, *Journal of Epidemiology and Community Health 39*, 1–8.

Gilbert, G. M., Arber, S., Byrne, J. D., and Dale, A. (1983) *General Household Survey 1980, SPSSx Version*, London: National Children's Bureau.

Gillies, P. (1987) Health Behaviour and health promotion in youth. In this volume.

Gove, W. R. (1973) Sex, marital status, and mortality, *American Journal of Sociology*, 79 (1), 45–67.

Gove, W. R. and Hughes, M. (1979) Possible causes for the apparent sex differences in physical health: an empirical investigation, *American Sociological Review, 44* (1), 126–46.

Greater Glasgow Health Board (1986) *Standardised Mortality Ratio for Subdivisions of Greater Glasgow. Maps for all Causes and Selected Causes of Death 1980_1982*, Information Services Department.

Hart, N. (1986) Inequalities in health: the individual versus the environment, *Journal of the Royal Statistical Society 149* (3), 228–46.

Illsley, R. (1955) Social class selection and class differences in relation to stillbirth and infant deaths, *British Medical Journal, 253*, 1520.

Illsley, R. (1986) Occupational class, selection and the production of inequalities in health, *Quarterly Journal of Social Affairs, 2* (2), 151–65.

Kessler, I. I. and Levin, M. I. (eds) (1970) *The Community as an Epidemiologic Laboratory: A Casebook of Community Studies*, Baltimore: Johns Hopkins University Press.

Koos, E. (1954) *The Health of Regionville: What People Said, Thought and Did About It*, New York: Hefner Publishing.

Lancet, Editorial (1985) Another Look at the Pill and Breast Cancer, *Lancet, ii*, 985–87.

Lundberg, O. (1986) Class and health: comparing Britain and Sweden, *Social Science and Medicine, 23* (5), 511.

Macintyre, S. (1986a) The patterning of health by social position in contemporary Britain: directions for sociological research, *Social Science and Medicine, 23* (4), 393–415

Macintyre, S. (1986b) *West of Scotland Twenty-07 Study; Physical Measures of Health, Development and Functioning*, MRC Medical Sociology Unit Working Paper No.3.

MacIver, S. (1988) (forthcoming) *West of Scotland Twenty-07 Study; Selection Criteria for the Region and Localities*, MRC Medical Sociology Unit Working Paper No. 4.

Marmot, M. and McDowell, M. (1986) Mortality decline and widening social inequalities, *Lancet*, 2nd Aug., 274–76.

Morgan, D. (1986) Gender, in R. Burgess (ed.), *Key Variables in Social Investigation*, London: RKP.

Nathanson, C. A. (1977) Sex, illness and medical care: a review of data, theory and method, *Social Science and Medicine, 11* (1), 13–25.

Parker, S. (1980) *Older Workers and Retirement*, London: HMSO.

Plant, M. A., Peck, D. F., Samnel, E. (1985) *Alcohol, Drugs and School Leavers*, London: Tavistock.

Royal College of General Practitioners, OPCS, DHSS (1986) *Morbidity Statistics from General Practice 1981–82*, London: HMSO.

Strathclyde Regional Council (1987) *Strathclyde Economic Trends No.17*, Chief Executive's Office.

Townsend, P. and Davidson, N. (1982) *Inequalities in Health: The Black Report*, Harmondsworth: Penguin.

Veness, J. (1962) *School-Leavers*, London: Methuen.

Verbrugge, L. (1983) Multiple roles and physical health of men and women, *Journal of Health and Social Behaviour*, *24* (1), 16–30.

West, P. (1986) *West of Scotland Twenty-07 Study: The Study of Youth and Health*, MRC Medical Sociology Unit Working Paper No.2.

West, P. (In press) Inequalities? Social class differentials in health in youth. *Social Science and Medicine*.

Whitehead, M. (1987) *The Health Divide: Inequalities in Health in the 1980s*, London: Health Education Council.

Wilkinsons, R. G. (1986) Occupational class, selection and inequalities in health: a reply to Raymond Illsley, *Quarterly Journal of Social Affairs*, *2* (4), 415–22.

7

CHRISTINA R. VICTOR

HEALTH INEQUALITY IN LATER LIFE:
AGE, GENDER OR CLASS?

The World Health Organisation declaration of 'Health For All by
the Year 2000' is a challenge to governments throughout the world
to improve the health status of their populations. One important
aspect of the Health For All (HFA) approach is the reduction of
inequalities in health status within populations. Such inequalities
may be focused around the concepts of age, class, ethnicity or
gender; or indeed some combination of these dimensions.

Inequalities in health status centred around the concept of social
class are the enduring pervasive feature of British society. Both
the Black Report (DHSS, 1980) and the Health Divide (HEC,
1987) have indicated that the health experience of the population
varies significantly with social class. A major longitudinal study
sponsored by OPCS study (Fox and Goldblatt, 1982) has confirmed the persistence and reality of class-based health inequalities
within the British population.

However, the debate about inequalities in health, especially
that focusing upon a class-based analysis, has largely concentrated
upon the population of working age. Rarely has this analysis been
extended to the population over retirement age. This is a significant
omission, as 17 per cent of the British population, approximately
9 million people, are now over statutory retirement age; 60 for
women and 65 for men. This apparent neglect of the analysis of
social class in the experience of ageing, especially in terms of
health status, reflects a naïve assumption upon the part of many
gerontologists that the major dimensions of stratification are not
important in old age. A second assumption is also involved which

75

is the stereotypical representation of later life as a time in which universal and inevitable biological decline manifests itself. Because all the elderly are assumed to be experiencing bad health there is no need to look for inequalities.

Too often gerontologists have looked at ageing in terms of the adjustment required between the individual and society, as in activity or disengagement theory (Marshall, 1987). Only recently have gerontologists considered how society and its systems of stratification influence and constrain the experience of old age. Phillips (1982) has argued that old age can only be understood by examining it in terms of social class.

This paper considers social class-based inequalities in health in old age using a variety of sources of data includng the General Household Survey (GHS) and a survey of the elderly under-taken by the author and colleagues in South Wales. Age- and gender-based inequalities are also examined.

Measuring health status

Typically, discussions of health inequalities are focused around mortality as, in Britain, these data are readily obtainable via the analysis of death certificates. Whilst mortality data are useful for making crude comparisons between different groups or areas, this is a highly limited conceptualisation of the notion 'health'. The use of mortality as a surrogate health indicator is predicted upon the assumption that the causes of mortality and morbidity in the population are synonymous. This is a questionable assumption for older age groups where the major sources of morbidity are chronic, long-term conditions which result in few deaths. Thus morbidity data are also used in this paper to provide a broader approach and definition to the study of inequalities in health. Several aspects of morbidity, including acute and chronic sickness, functional disabil-ity, mental status, incontinence and difficulties with sight/hearing, are employed. In addition perceived health status is also included in the analysis.

Method

Two main sources of data are used in this paper. The first data set is the 1980 General Household Survey (GHS). The GHS is a continuous survey of a random sample of the population of Great Britain resident in private households. This survey has taken place annually since 1971. In 1980 100,000 households were selected to participate in the study, 16 per cent of whom declined to take part or were not contacted. The GHS always includes a broad range of subject areas including occupation, health, housing and income. In addition the 1980 GHS included a series of supplementary questions for people aged 65 and over which related to physical disability, use of community services and the receipt of informal care.

The 1980 GHS includes questions about morbidity, both acute episodes of ill health within the 14 days prior to interview and long-standing disability which imposes a restriction on the respondent's lifestyle. Also included in the GHS are questions relating to sight and hearing problems as well as an overall question relating to subjects' overall perceived health status.

The 1980 GHS also included a series of questions about respondents' ability to perform a series of six tasks. These tasks are drawn from the disability index described by Townsend (1979). This is a well validated and reliable measure which has been used in previous studies of the elderly (Bond and Carstairs, 1982). The index describes the ability of subjects to perform a series of tasks considered essential to an independent life in the community such as cooking, self-care and house-care. Tasks which are performed unaided are scored 0, those done with assistance score 1 and those which cannot be undertaken score 2. Six of the original nine tasks are included in the 1980 GHS giving the score a possible range of 0-12. Following Bebbington's (1982) typology a score of 0 is classed as not disabled, 1 to 2 are mildly disabled, 3 to 6 as moderately disabled and 7 and over as severely disabled.

The second data set is derived from a study in South Wales which evaluated the effectiveness of health visitors working with the elderly (Vetter, 1986). A random sample of elderly persons aged 70 and over living at home in two areas of Wales, one urban and one rural, was selected from the age-sex registers of two general practices. Response rates of 95 per cent were obtained giving a total sample of 2,500. Data were collected about social class via a series of questions about occupation. The questionnaire data included detailed information about various aspects of morbidity. Only the data relating to mental status and incontinence are reported here. Three measures of mental status are described – anxiety, depression and memory loss.

This analysis uses a gradational approach to the definition of social class using occupation as the defining variables. There are a number of limitations inherent in this approach (Victor and Evandrou, 1987). However, the five-fold typology of class used by the Registrar General is currently the most widely used and readily available means of measuring class. Indeed it may be that this is more appropriate for older people than some other status

Table 7.1. Standardised mortality of males by
social class in England and Wales

	AGE		
	15–64	65–74	75+
Class I	66	68	73
Class II	77	81	84
Class IIIn	105	86	92
Class IIIm	96	100	105
Class IV	109	106	108
Class V	124	109	116

Source: Fox *et al.* (1985), table 2.

variables suggested for younger age groups, such as car ownership
and tenure.

Results

Mortality. When analysing mortality data for the elderly we must
be aware of the limitations imposed upon this type of analysis by
inaccuracy in the certification of the cause of death amongst the
older age groups.

In the majority of deaths which occur annually in Great Britain,
78 per cent are of people over 65 years of age. The death rate
increased sharply with age. At all ages over 65 years, female death
rates are substantially lower than those for males.

In Britain, deaths are not equally distributed throughout the
calendar year. McDowell (1981) reports that, for all age groups,
there is a marked seasonality in the death rate, with a considerable
excess of deaths during the winter months. This seasonal excess of
deaths is most marked amongst the elderly population. This marked
seasonal variation in death rate is not a feature of other countries
of Western Europe, many of which experience considerably more
severe winters than Britain.

There are substantial variations in death rates between the
standard statistical regions. Death rates for the elderly are highest
amongst the regions of the north and west compared with the south
and east. In the East Anglia region males in the 65 to 74 age group
have a death rate of 40 per 1,000 compared with 52 per 1,000 for
the same age group in the north. Similar gradients in death rates
between the regions are characteristic of females. However, the
gradient in death rates between regions is less marked for females as

compared with males. At all ages, however, females display lower death rates than males. This pattern of geographical variations in mortality for the elderly mirrors regional variations in mortality and morbidity characteristic of younger age groups (Townsend and Davidson, 1982).

Table 1 demonstrates that, for males over the age of 65, there is a strong class-based gradient in mortality which mirrors that characteristic of younger age groups. Consistently, the elderly who were employed in professional occupations demonstrate a lower mortality rate than their counterparts who were engaged in manual occupations. Thus, males from manual occupations demonstrate a mortality rate which is 60 per cent higher than that of their counterparts from the professional classes.

Morbidity. Some of the most commonly used measures relate to the incidence of limiting illness amongst the population. These indicators usually differentiate between acute health problems and those of a more long standing or chronic nature. Acute health problems are usually defined as self-limiting conditions of short duration, usually three months or less. Included under this heading are such conditions as colds, influenza or accidental injuries. Usually acute illnesses are characterised by symptoms or causes for which medical techniques or other forms of intervention may effect a cure.

Each year the General Household Survey asks its respondents about acute health problems which have restricted their normal level of activity in the 14 days before interview. Using these data, there is an increase in the fraction of subjects reporting an acute illness with age. In the 16–44 age range, 10 per cent of males reported suffering from an acute illness episode compared with 17 per cent of those aged over 75. At all ages females consistently report a higher level of acute illness than males. However, it is important to keep these data in context. Even in the very oldest age groups, acute illness only affects 20 per cent of males and 25 per cent of females; the rest remaining free of such health problems.

At all ages the prevalence of acute illness is slightly higher amongst females as compared with males. The prevalence of acute illness varies with the social class of the older person; 14 per cent of elderly in social classes I and II experienced acute health problems in the 14 days before interview compared with 18 per cent of those from social classes IV and V. This trend was not, however, statistically significant.

In addition to being asked if they have suffered an acute illness episode, the General Household Survey asks respondents to state the duration (in days) that it restricted their normal activities.

Males in the 16–44 age range experience limited activity because of acute health problems for an average of 15.6 days a year compared with 45.6 days for males aged over 75. For these types of illnesses, older people's activity levels are influenced for much longer than younger subjects. Again at all ages females have a higher average number of restricted activity days than males. There was no significant difference between the social classes in the average number of days of restricted activity for older people.

Chronic health problems are, by definition, long-term and not usually characterised by a cure. Medical intervention may (or may not) alleviate some, or all, of the associated symptoms. Examples of such long-term health problems are multiple sclerosis and arthritis. It is these types of health problems which are specifically associated by both the general public and many professional health workers alike as being an integral, inevitable and universal feature of old age.

The proportion of the population which reports that they have a long-standing illness or disability increases sharply with age. A quarter of males and females in the 16–44 age group report that they have a long-standing illness compared with at least 60 per cent of the over 75 age group. Only for the older age groups is there any difference in the reported prevalence of long-standing illness between the sexes.

The existence of long-standing illness or disability may not, however, impair the activity levels or lifestyle of the sufferer. The popular stereotype of old age as a time of universal and inevitable chronic health and impaired activity is far from correct. Whilst the prevalence of a long-standing limiting illness increases with age it is not a universal characteristic of later life. Almost half the men and women aged over 80 years of age do not have a long-standing disability or illness which impairs their activity levels. Amongst the elderly, limiting long-standing disability rates are higher for females than males.

The percentage of older people reporting that they experience a long-standing, limiting disability varies with social class from 37 per cent of those from a professional occupation background to 47 per cent from the semi-skilled and unskilled occupation groups (Table 2).

Functional capacity. Another way of looking at chronic health problems has been via the collection of data about the ability of the elderly to undertake a variety of activities and tasks considered essential to an independent life in the community. These research instruments are loosely grouped together as measures of functional

Table 7.2. Health status of the elderly person by their social class (%)

Health	I & II	IIIn	IIIm	IV & V	Total
		SOCIAL CLASS			
Limiting longstanding illness	37	41	46	47	44
Total	(511)	(1,056)	(961)	(1,664)	(4,192)
Acute illness	14	17	16	18	17
Total	(513)	(1,057)	(964)	(1,668)	(4,202)
Slight difficulty	21	24	24	27	25
Total	(490)	(1,022)	(914)	(1,599)	(4,025)
Hearing difficulty	34	30	35	32	33
Total	(489)	(1,024)	(916)	(1,605)	(4,034)

capacity. A large number of these measures have been devised. Typical of these measures of functional capacity is that described by Townsend (1979). This has been used in a large number of community studies of the elderly population (Bond and Carstairs, 1982; Vetter *et al.*, 1984a). The nine items included in his list of activities cover all the different types of physical function the elderly might be expected to undertake when living at home such as bending, lifting, carrying and reaching. This is essentially a dictionary approach in which the ability of the older person to undertake a series of tasks is recorded upon a check-list.

Collecting data about such activities of daily living (often referred to in the literature as ADL) does pose some difficulties for the researcher. Asking the older person to perform these tasks, such as making a cup of tea, in a test setting in a hospital may reproduce artificially high or low results. Collecting the data in an interview situation presents problems of sex bias. Survey work undertaken by the author and others in Wales encountered problems in getting older males to respond to questions about their ability to perform tasks such as ironing or cooking. Although many of the males interviewed were healthy and active, they almost universally reported that they could not possibly do the ironing for that was seen as the job of their wife.

Given these limitations, Table 3 describes the ability of a sample of the over 70s in Wales to perform the nine activities included in the Townsend index. The majority of older people can undertake these activities without difficulty; only a minority are unable to undertake these tasks without the assistance of another person.

One cannot assume that an age-related increase in disability implies that older people cannot manage to care for themselves

Table 7.3. Ability of the elderly to undertake self-care
and housecare tasks (%)

| | DIFFICULTY | | |
Activity	None	Some	Unable alone
Washing all over	87	7	6
Cutting toenails	64	17	19
Catching a bus	77	8	15
Going up and down stairs	77	16	8
Heavy housework	68	16	17
Going shopping	62	14	24
Cooking a meal	87	5	8
Reaching a shelf	73	12	15
Tying a knot	94	4	2

Source: Research Team for the Care of the Elderly
unpublished data.

adequately in their homes. Despite often severe limitations of activity, most older people develop coping strategies and modify their lifestyle to take into account these restrictions. This adaptation strategy is not unique to the elderly but rather applies generally to all those who experience long-term health problems.

As with acute illness and long-standing, limiting disability, functional capacity demonstrates a relationship with the social class of the older person. The elderly from professional and managerial occupations are less likely to be classified as disabled than their counterparts from manual occupations. Thus 60 per cent of elderly from classes I and II were defined as not disabled compared with 45 per cent of classes IV and V. The fraction defined as severely disabled does not seem to vary with social class; rather it is the lesser categories of disability which seem to vary most markedly with the occupational status of the older person.

Problems with sight and hearing. Problems with sight and hearing. A further dimension of health status related to the special senses of sight and hearing. The proportion of people who experience difficulties with either sight or hearing increases substantially with age. There are good biological explanations for the age-related deteriorations in the functioning of the senses of sight and hearing.

Unlike the distribution of chronic illness, there is no clear relationship with gender. Older women are more likely to experience

Table 7.4. Subjective health rating by age and sex (%)

	65–69		70–74		75–79		80–84		85+	
	m	f	m	f	m	f	m	f	m	f
Good	67	61	61	57	60	56	63	61	63	69
Fair	27	31	30	36	31	35	30	30	28	25
Poor	6	7	9	7	9	9	7	8	9	7

Source: Bond and Carstairs (1982), table 23.

sight difficulties with age than men whilst the opposite relationship is evident for hearing difficulties. Again, however, we should be wary of perceiving old age as a time of universal deterioration of the special senses. Even amongst the very oldest age groups difficulties with sight and hearing are reported by only half of these age groups. There is no relationship between difficulties with sight and hearing and social class.

Incontinence. Incontinence is an aspect of health in later life which has received much less attention than, for example, functional capacity or mental status, for it still remains rather a taboo subject. The causes of incontinence may be both social or physical (or a combination of both). Whatever the causes, the results can be profound for the older person, causing strain amongst carers, preventing admission to sheltered housing, residential accommodation, and restricting the social activities of the sufferer.

Establishing the prevalence of incontinence amongst the elderly (or any other part of the population) presents difficulties for the researcher. First, we must define what constitutes incontinence and the degree of severity of the affliction. Second, in interviews sufferers may be reluctant to admit to this problem because of its extreme negative connotations. Data gathered in interview surveys may, therefore, substantially underestimate the true prevalence of incontinence within the population. Whilst there are substantial variations in prevalences between studies, the data are consistent in indicating that this is a problem which is more common amongst females than males.

Subjective health status. Another approach towards the measurement of health status is to record the perception the individual has of his or her health. Many health status surveys of the population ask respondents to evaluate their health as good, fair or poor in the last year (or a specified period before the interview).

Compared with younger age groups the elderly, of either sex,

Table 7.5. Subjective health status by social class (%)

General health (in last year)	SOCIAL CLASS				
	I & II	IIIn	IIIm	IV & V	Total
Good	49	43	34	31	37
Fairly good	35	37	42	42	40
Poor	16	20	25	28	24
Total	(489)	(1,022)	(918)	(1,605)	(4,034)

are more likely to rate their health as fair or not good (Table 4). Given the increased prevalence of chronic illness with age this is not surprising. Perhaps more surprising is that so few elderly rate their health as 'not good' in the face of the high incidence of chronic illness and impairments which afflict them. This anomaly probably reflects the highly subjective way we define and evaluate our own health status.

Older people display a high degree of realism when evaluating their own health. Like any other group they will evaluate their own health status with reference to that of their peers rather than to either other age groups or some hypothetical achievable 'best' state. If we ask people to rate their health as good, fair or poor for their age, we can see from Table 4 that there is remarkably little alteration in responses with age.

As with the other dimensions of health status, perceived health shows a relationship with social class. Table 5 demonstrates that elderly from the professional and managerial groups are more likely to rate their health as good than their counterparts from manual occupations. The opposite pattern is evident for the fraction of older people rating their health as poor. Almost a half of the elderly in the professional occupation groups rate their health as good compared with 30 per cent of those elderly from the unskilled and semi-skilled occupation groups.

Mental health. Organic states are often referred to as senility, a term which is both inaccurate and emotive, and implies that progressive deterioration, which accompanies the disorder, is a normal part of ageing. It cannot be stressed too strongly that organic brain syndromes are not part of normal ageing but a specific disease process which, as yet, we cannot treat or reverse. Functional or affective disorders comprise a variety of states such as anxiety, depression and disturbances of mood.

Women are more likely to be classified as suffering from an

Table 7.6. Prevalence of mental disorder by social
class (%)

	SOCIAL CLASS			
	I & II	IIIn	IIIm	IV & V
Dementia	7	5	4	8
Anxiety	9	13	14	19
Depression	3	7	6	7

affective disorder than men (Vetter *et al.*, 1984). There was no
sex difference in the prevalence of organic states and there is only
a marginal increase in reported prevalence with age (Bond and
Carstairs, 1982). It seems that it is fairly rare for a clinical affective
disorder to manifest itself for the first time in old age. The majority
of psychiatric disorders are usually found in older people who have
had a history of this type of problem in earlier life.

No relationship was observed between social class and the prevalence of dementia or depression. However, Table 6 indicates that
anxiety was significantly related to the social class of the older
person.

Discussion

Old age is a stage in the life-cycle about which there are numerous stereotypes. To present an overstatement of commonly held
beliefs, the old are portrayed as dependent and characterised by
a lack of social autonomy. They are neglected by their family and
friends and pose a threat to the living standards of younger age
groups by being a 'burden' which consumes without producing.
The elderly are perceived as a single homogeneous group and
the experience of ageing is characterised as being the same for all
individuals, irrespective of their circumstances.

The debate about inequalities in health has, in Britain, largely
ignored the older ages. This reflects the prevalence of two stereotypes. The first, noted above, is that the experience of ageing is
very similar for all old people. The second assumption reflects the
influence of the bio-medical model in the study of ageing. Old age
is presented as a time of universal and inevitable biological decline.
Thus old age is portrayed as a time when ill health is the norm. Consequently the study of inequalities in health status is irrelevant.

Three dimensions of differentiation were presented in this
paper: age, gender and class. Due to the size of the data set,

it was not possible to consider other important dimensions of differentiation such as ethnicity.

Social class is an important dimension of differentiation within British society (Reid 1977). Its importance in the experience of old age is increasingly being recognised, with researchers looking at how the major dimensions of stratification explain and influence the experience of later life. The paper has used data from two major sources to consider the presence of health inequalities amongst older people. This challenges the stereotypes of the elderly as being indifferentiated and as being characterised by universal physical and mental ill-health.

The definition and conceptualisation of health is both culturally and temporally specific. Translating these concepts into operational measures which can be systematically applied across populations is problematic. Thus, measures of the health of populations can take a variety of different forms. Typically, studies which have investigated inequalities in health have tended to concentrate upon describing differences in health status. Given the greatly increased prevalence of chronic illness in old age, it seemed appropriate, in this study, to focus upon measures of morbidity.

This research has distinguished between several different types of morbidity. First a distinction has been made between acute and chronic illness. Whilst there is an important difference between these two types of morbidity, it is important not to think of these two groups as being totally distinct and separate.

Both age and gender were important sources of differences in health status amongst older people. However, these difference were only observed for the chronic health problems. Acute health status showed little variation with either age or sex. Although the prevalence of chronic, physical ill-health increased with age, it was not, even in the oldest age groups, the norm. Thus these data show that the stereotype of later life as a time of universal ill health is inaccurate.

Fox *et al.* (1985) have described a substantial social, class-based variation in mortality for males over retirement age. This differential was only observed for four morbidity measures; chronic illness, disability, urinary incontinence and anxiety. In addition, subject health status was also related to class. These relationships were independent of the influence of age or gender.

Explaining why some, but not all, morbidity measures showed a significant variation with class is problematic. Like younger age groups the elderly from classes IV and V have substantially higher prevalence of chronic illness than their counterparts from classes I and II. However, this differential is lower than that characteristic of mortality. Disability was also significantly differentiated by social class. Thus it seems that, as far as long-standing chronic illness/disablement are concerned, social class is an important variable and the higher prevalence of these disorders amongst the elderly from non-manual backgrounds reflects the culmination of a lifetime of disadvantage and inequality.

Incontinence is a particular problem for older people because it is a medical condition which has profound social implications for the sufferer. That incontinence is differentially distributed throughout the elderly in terms of age and sex has been noted elsewhere (Vetter *et al.*, 1984). However, a social class variation has never been previously reported. It is difficult to decide from these data whether this is simply an artefact produced by the data or represents a 'true' difference in the health experience of older people. It is possible that response bias, brought about by the tendency for non-manual elderly to under-report their incontinence, may have produced these data. Alternatively, there may be a differential class response by service providers to the problem of incontinence resulting in the problem being more effectively treated in elderly from professional backgrounds.

It is not surprising that dementia does not show a relationship with social class and nothing in the suggested aetiology of the disease is related to class. Anxiety and depression seem, however, to be more causally related to individual's social environment. The social-class variation in anxiety levels may reflect differences in their experience of later life which might influence anxiety such as housing or financial circumstances, whereas the major sources of depression such as bereavement may be more equally distributed throughout later life.

Inequalities in health status are a feature of old age, as indeed they are of other stages in the life-cycle. However, the services provided for older people do not seem to be positively attempting to reduce the identified inequalities. Consequently, policy makers need to be made aware of the profound differences in health status within the elderly population and to develop ways to combat them.

Acknowledgements

I would like to thank the Office of Population Censuses and Surveys (OPCS), who carry out the General Household Survey, for allowing me to use the data, and also the ESRC data archive for preparing and distributing the data. The analysis was facilitated by the use of SIR files prepared at the University of Surrey by G. N. Gilbert, A. Dale, S. Arber and J. O'Byrne.

The 1980 GHS file used in the analysis was created by M. Evandrou.

My thanks also to the St. Mary's Hospital Special Trustees for financial support.

References

Bebbington, A. (1982) *Using the GHS as the basis for territorial indicators of need amongst the elderly*, Personal Social Services Research Unit, University of Kent.

Bond, J. and Carstairs, V. (1982) *The Elderly in Clackmannan*, Scottish Health Services Studies No. 42, Scottish Home and Health Department, Edinburgh.

Department of Health and Social Security (1980) *Inequalities in Health (The Black Report)*, HMSO.

Fox, J. and Goldblatt, P. (1982) *The Longitudinal Study: Socio-demographic morality differentials*, OPCS, HMSO.

Fox, J., Jones, D., Moser, K., Goldblatt, P. (1985) Socio-economic differences in mortality, *Population Trends*, 40, 10-16.

Health Education Council (1986) *The Health Divide*, London: HEC.

Marshall, V. W. (ed.) (1987) *Later Life: The Social Psychology of Ageing*, Sage.

Phillip, C. (1982) *Capitalism and the Construction of Old Age*, London: Metheun.

Reid, I. (1977) *Social Class Differences in Britain*, London: Fontana.

Townsend, P. (1979) *Poverty in the United Kingdom*, Harmondsworth: Penguin.

Townsend, P. and Davidson, N. (1981) *The Black Report*, Harmondsworth: Penguin.

Vetter, N. J. (1986) The measurement of psychological problems in the elderly in general practice, *International Journal of Geriatric Psychiatry*, 1, 127-34.

Vetter, N. J., Jones, D. A., Victor, C. R. (1984) The effectiveness of health visitors working with the elderly in general practice, *British Medical Journal*, 288, 369-72.

Victor, C. R. and Evandrou, M. (1987) Does social class matter in later life, *Proceedings of the 1986 BSG Conference*, London: Croom Helm (forthcoming).

8

JENNIE POPAY AND MEL BARTLEY

CONDITIONS OF LABOUR AND WOMEN'S HEALTH

In recent years there has been a surge of interest amongst researchers, policy makers and health care professionals in the health experience of people in different social classes (Whitehead, 1987). To a lesser extent, though still notable, there has also been a growth of interest in the different health experiences of men and women. Lois Verbrugge (1985) describes these gender inequalities as an iceberg of ill health. The top of this iceberg, she argues, is a deeply masculine hue, with men more likely to die prematurely and to experience life threatening illnesses. The bottom, however, the great invisible bulk of the iceberg, is a strong female hue, for it is women who experience the most ill health. In essence then, it can be argued that whilst women get quantity of life years, men get the quality.

In seeking to identify the aetiological factors generating inequalities in health, research has followed many different lines of enquiry, though a concern with individual behaviour has dominated. There are, however, important differences between research concerned with social class and that concerned with gender-related inequalities in health.

Research on social class inequalities, for instance, is concerned above all with differential mortality experience – primarily of men (Wilkinson, 1986). There has been an important and influential – albeit limited – tradition of research focusing on the aetiological significance of people's public lives in paid work and of the material conditions in which they live and work. This is reflected in the pervasive use of occupation as a measure of social class and in studies of specific occupational hazards, and of the health consequences of poor housing and low income (Fox and Goldblatt, 1982; Martin *et al.*, 1987; Marmot *et al.*, 1984).

In contrast, research on gender inequalities has been concerned above all with the morbidity experience of women. Here, research deviating from the dominant individualistic mode has focused on the private world of the family and on the social, rather than the material dimensions of this sphere (Verbrugge, 1985).

This division in research on social class and gender inequalities in health has serious consequences for our understanding of aetiology in relation to women's experience of health and illness for it has led to a neglect of the health implications of the material conditions of women's lives and of their unpaid labour in the home.

Research on social class inequalities, for example, consistently fails to use measures sensitive to material disadvantage amongst women. First, occupationally based measures of social class are constructed from a classification of occupations which are predominantly male and which are therefore insensitive to the differences in women's occupations. Second, such measures cannot locate an increasing number of people, large numbers of them women, who depend *in the long term* on the social security system or on a partner for their financial support. Third, they are a very crude measure of individual living standards, unable to deal with the possibility of unequal access to resources *within* households. Finally, research focusing on the public world of paid employment does not and cannot offer insights into the health implications of conditions in the private world of the family. Research on gender inequalities in health does not provide a compensatory balance. Here as we have already suggested, the focus has been on women's *social* role in the family and on the different socialisation of women compared to men. Together, it is argued, these aspects of women's lives 'allow' them to adopt the sick role more often than men and to be ready to report ill health. Neglected is the possibility that women may really be sicker than men and that the demands of their domestic labour and the material conditions they labour in, may make a major contribution to their experience of ill health (Gove and Hughes, 1981).

In essence the problem is that health researchers have not taken the sexual division of labour seriously enough. The important word here is *labour*. According to data from a recent survey of 1,700 households in London, women with children spend on average 64 hours a week on domestic labour if they have a full time paid job, 75 hours a week if they have a part-time paid job and 87 hours a week if they have no paid job (Kowarzik and Popay). In total 57 per cent of the women in this sample 'laboured' in the home for at least 5 hours a day compared to 14 per cent of men. Given the scale of this labour it would seem to be important that research concerned to explain women's experience of ill health in different social classes and compared to men, should treat the home as a work-place. It is a work-place which disproportionately 'employs' women and in which workers may be exposed to a range of physical, chemical and psychological health hazards, *comparable to, not different from* those identified in the formal labour market.

Despite the limitations and gender blindness of existing research on the health implications of formal labour, this work does provide concepts and theoretical frameworks with which to begin to re-define labour conditions to include women's unpaid work. Essentially, there are two fields of enquiry to which we can turn: that concerned with the material conditions of paid employment and that concerned with the psycho-social conditions. Looking at the literature in these two spheres it is possible to illustrate 1) how the concepts used may be extended to provide research tools applicable to both domestic and paid labour and 2) how a more coherent theory of the relationship between labour conditions and social class and gender inequalities in health might be developed.

Measuring domestic labour conditions

Amongst the most innovative recent contribution to research on the relationship between social class inequalities in health and the material conditions of labour is Peter Townsend's work on the concept of 'Occupational Deprivation' (Townsend, 1979). The index he has been constructing has five main dimensions: income from work, the relative severity of the job, the security of the job, the conditions and amenities at work and fringe benefits attaching to the job. Transferring elements of this index to the domestic sphere presents formidable difficulties, but it also raises important questions about the way in which the concept is being elaborated and operationalised in the formal labour market. Take income for example. Is it possible to transfer a concept of income from work to the domestic sector? One could simply argue that those in the domestic sector simply do not 'earn' an income. But this is not strictly accurate. What of child benefit, housekeeping allowances, state benefits to women not in employment and state payments to foster parents? Exploring this issue forces one to consider exactly what it is about income that is important in relation to health inequalities. Access to resources for personal consumption or for collective consumption? Access to a means of control and a source of power? Such questions also have implications for the measures of income used in relation to the formal labour market.

Perhaps the most straightforward example of the way in which a concept of occupational deprivation might be extended to the domestic sphere is provided by measures of conditions and amenities at work. Using data from the recent survey of London households referred to earlier we have been able to look at the labour conditions of men and women in the formal and the domestic sector in relation to six of Townsend's indices: air pollution, noise, damp, temperature extremes, access to a lavatory and access to first-aid facilities.

This survey was not designed to explore conditions of domestic labour and the variables available for use relating to this sphere left much to be desired. Questions on noise in the domestic sphere, for instance, did not specifically ask about the noise of children. Similarly, in relation to temperature extremes the variable we used for domestic labour involved the response to a question about the number of rooms heated at least once during a day. This is likely to be an underestimate of women's exposure to cold in the home, for qualitative research suggests that in order to save money women will switch off heating during the day, heating the rooms when children and partners are at home (Graham, 1985; Adams *et al.*, 1969). Additionally, variables relating to the two spheres are not always directly comparable. Whilst people in paid work were asked if they had access to first-aid facilities, for example, the variable we used in relation to the domestic sector refers to whether people felt they had easy access to a general practitioner or an emergency hospital department.

Despite these difficulties and the fact that our analysis to date is extremely preliminary, the findings presented in Table 8.1 are of interest. As can be seen, on all dimensions except noise and access to first aid, women appear to 'labour' in more advantageous conditions in the formal sector than they do in the domestic sector.

Turning then to research on the psycho-social conditions of paid labour, research in this field has concentrated on concepts of 'stress'. Karasek and his colleagues have refined this notoriously

Table 8.1. Aspects of material conditions in the paid workplace and the home. Proportions exposed to various hazards

	Formal labour market only* (N=271)		Domestic labour only (N=325)	
Site of exposure:	*Paid workplace*		*Home*	
	Women N=58	Men N=213	Women N=316	Men N=9†
Percentage exposed to:				
Air pollution	17	33	29	—
Noise	34	51	29	—
Damp	10	25	29	—
Temperature extremes	8	9	33	—
No WC access	2	5	1	—
No first aid/clinic/hospital	4	7	7	—

* Less than 7 hours domestic work. † Numbers too small for analysis.

elusive idea into two dimensions: job demand (the psycho-social pressures involved in different forms of paid labour) and job decision latitude (the scope offered in a particular paid job for the individual to exercise autonomy and self-actualisation, as well as to adapt the pace of work according to their own discretion). In the existing literature job demand has been operationalised in terms of such features as the length of the working day, machine-pacing of work and 'problems' (not further specified) with superiors or workmates. Job-decision latitude is seen in terms of whether or not the worker is able to make or to receive private phone calls during the day, or leave work for short periods on private business.

One has only to itemise these measures to realise how difficult it is to devise appropriate measures of the wide variety of conditions under which people labour even in the formal sector of the economy. Nevertheless, it is possible to see how concepts of job demand and decision latitude viewed from a purely psycho-social perspective might be applied to domestic labour. One dimension explored by Karasek *et al.* (1981), for instance, is the extent to which a job is considered *hectic*. What could be more hectic than the demands of let us say two children under five years of age, a helpless partner combined with an absence of convenient, safe, play space and domestic appliances in good condition. This example not only illustrates how a concept might be transferred to the domestic sector but also how it might be operationalised. Job-decision latitude is similarly transferable. Take, for example, leaving the job for private business. Once again, it takes little imagination (at least for women) to see how little latitude there will be for private business – even for thinking one's own thoughts – for a woman living in the circumstances described above.

Towards an integrated theory of labour conditions and women's health

Research has demonstrated that the material conditions in which people live and work will have an effect, either positive or negative, on their experience of health and illness. Similarly, despite the fact that 'they may know not what they measure' researchers have identified a strong relationship between 'stressful' working conditions and adverse health outcomes. It is therefore obvious that the combined effects of material and psycho-social hazards of labour need to be taken into account in attempts to understand social class and gender inequalities in health. Additionally, as we have argued, it is important that researchers take into account the material and psycho–social conditions of women's unpaid labour in the home.

A beginning may be made in this endeavour by developing two new concepts – that of labour demand (rather than job-demand) and that of resolution latitude (rather than job-decision latitude). It is apparent to us that there are both material and psycho-social dimensions to each of these and that it is with regard to these two dimensions that we can begin to understand better the commonality of women's experience of ill health compared to men and the diverging experience of women in different social classes.

With regard to the material demands of domestic labour, for example, it is undisputably the case that poor women will be exposed to greater health hazards from damp and cold working conditions in the home, etc. than middle- and upper-class women. The psycho-social demands of domestic labour may, however, be more similar for women in different social classes. The emotional and physical demands of caring for children, which may well explain why women are more often ill than men, have been little documented in research, but there is a powerfully striking thread in the experience of these two women: one of them, Jane, alone with a child living on supplementary benefit, the other, Sara, living with

her husband and two children on an income in excess of £60,000
(Popay and Jones, 1987).

Jane:

'You've got to love and care for them, you've got to look after
them properly, making sure they're healthy . . . you can't just
walk away.'

Sara:

'It's a tremendous responsibility having children, bringing
them up in the best way that one can . . . I don't think
people who haven't got children actually understand what it's
like . . . You're not doing everything just for yourself, you are
doing everything at the back of your mind with the children in
mind. I know I run my life around them and I do very little I
want to do. . . .'

It is also probable that the material resources available to middle-
and upper-class women will allow them greater latitude to resolve
some of the demands of their domestic labour – the hiring of
nannies or other forms of child care, for instance, the purchase
of good quality household appliances, access to a car or the ability
to mobilise social support. However, again it may be the case
that across social classes, there are common psycho-social factors inhibiting women's latitude to resolve the demands of their
domestic labour. Of paramount importance here and distinguishing
domestic labour from much paid labour, is the strong sense of moral
obligation or personal responsibility that women feel in relation to
their role as mothers. Again, the similarities in the experience of
the two women quoted above are a powerful illustration of this
point:

Jane:

'I do think it's a lot more stressful than people realise being
a mother . . . Sometimes you just want to scream and say
I can't stand it any more. And I do, I just cry . . . I don't
really ever get a break. It's just 100 per cent of the time,
you can't be ill, you have to get up, you have to carry on
. . . when they start talking they go on and on and when
they see you sit down they say "can I have a drink" . . .
not being able to have the freedom to walk down the road,
I mean that sounds pathetic, but there's a lot of pressure,
I don't really relax unless she's asleep or something like
that.'

Sara:

'I think . . . by the end of the day when you would like
to have some time for your husband or for oneself you're

actually too physically exhausted to do anything. I went away
for a few days about 6 months ago and it was just wonderful
to have time to sit down and talk without being interrupted,
that was the first thing, and to eat a meal without sort of
thinking you have to get up . . . I think that one forgets
how much time they actually take up in a complete day
and I think we still need time as adults and its difficult, it's
very difficult to find it . . . the tiredness . . . the exhaustion.'

Theoretically then, it can be argued that there are strong common
strands across social classes in women's experience of domestic
labour – in terms of the psycho-social aspects of the demands of
this labour and the latitude they have to resolve such demands.
These common experiences may well 'explain' it in terms of their
being more often ill rather than more likely to report being ill!
Conversely, the material conditions of domestic labour for women
in different social classes and their differential access to resources
to resolve the physical demands of this labour, can be argued to
be an important influence on social class patterns of mortality and
morbidity amongst women. Such a theoretical perspective is also
consistent with the patterns of mortality identified amongst women
in the OPCS longitudinal study. These data suggest that the mortality gradient is in fact steeper between full-time housewives assigned
to social classes using their partners' occupations than amongst
women in paid employment assigned to social classes using their
own occupation (Moser *et al.*, 1987).

What we are proposing then is a model of the relationship
between labour conditions and inequalities in health which incorpor-
ates a concern with both the material and psycho-social conditions
of labour and the interaction between these two dimensions, and a
concern with both paid and unpaid labour. We have focused much
of our discussion on domestic labour. However, we have also
suggested that exploring how existing concepts of job demand and
decision latitude might be applied to the domestic sphere may also
point to limitations in the way they are being applied in research on
paid labour. Finally, the approach we are suggesting would allow
direct comparisons of the health implications of conditions in the
two spheres of labour as well as allowing researchers to take into
account the involvement of many individuals – most of them women
– in both paid and unpaid labour.

References

Adams, B., Ash, J., Littlewood, J. (1969) *The Family at Home: A Study of Households in Sheffield*, HMSO.
Fox, A. J. and Goldblatt, P. O. (1982) *Longitudinal Study: Socio-demographic mortality differentials 1971–75 England and Wales*, HMSO.
Gove, W. and Hughes, M. (1981) Beliefs vs data: more on the illness behaviour of men and women, *Amer. Soc. Review.*, 46, 123–8.
Graham, H. (1985) Caring for the Family, Unpublished research report later abridged version published as HEC Research Report No.1.
Karasek, R., Baker, D., Maxer, F., Ahlbom, A., Theorell, T., (1981) Job-decision, job demands and cardiovascular disease: a prospective study of Swedish men. *Amer. J. of Pub. Hlth.*, 71, 694–705.
Kowarzik, U., and Popay, J. Unpublished analysis of data from the London Living Standards Survey produced by Ute Kowarzik and forthcoming in a paper on Women's Unpaid Work.
Marmot, M. G., Shipley, M. J., Rose, G. (1984) Inequalities in health – specific explanations or a general pattern? *Lancet, 1,* 1003–6.
Martin, C. J., Platt, S. D., Hunt, S. M. (1987) Housing conditions and ill-health, *BMJ, 294,* 1125–7.
Moser, K., Pugh, H., Goldblatt, P. (1987) Inequalities in women's health: developing an alternative approach, City University, Social Statistics Research Unit, LS Working Paper No 54.
Popay, J. and Jones, G. (1987) *Women's Health in Households with Dependent Children*, Paper presented to annual conference of the Women's Medical Federation.
Townsend, P. (1979) *Poverty in the United Kingdom*, Harmondsworth: Penguin.
Whitehead, M. (1987) *The Health Divide: Inequalities in Health in the 1980s*, London: Health Education Council.
Wilkinson, R. G. (1986) Income and mortality, in R. G. Wilkinson (ed.), *Class and Health: Research and Longitudinal Data*, London: Tavistock.
Verbrugge, L. M. (1985) Gender and health: an update on hypotheses and evidence, *J. Health and Soc. Behav.*, 26, 156–82.

Personal Behaviour and the
Public Health

9

SONJA M. HUNT

THE PUBLIC HEALTH IMPLICATIONS
OF PRIVATE CARS

The current vogue for targeting individual behaviour as a major factor in the aetiology of disease and disability can be seen as an interesting example of the creation of social problems and the manipulation of public awareness. Primarily four types of behaviour receive a disproportionate amount of attention. These are smoking, dietary habits, exercise and alcohol consumption. Why these four should have been 'chosen' in preference to other, perhaps more pertinent, human activities is, of course, related to the fact that powerful groups, whether medical, educational or commercial have the capacity to influence the flow of information and debate on matters affecting the public health. Directing attention to some issues rather than others can be seen as part of the social construction of 'problems' whereby certain groups have the power to act collectively to define a problem and then initiate attempts to relieve, change or eliminate the problem (Kitsuse and Spector, 1975).

The implications of private car ownership for the public health have thus largely escaped serious attention, principally because there have been few people with any interest in raising it as an issue. This may be related to the fact that those people with the power to do so are themselves likely to have a 'lifestyle' in which the motor car plays a prominent role. There are political and economic reasons too. The road lobby is very powerful and enormous amounts of revenue are raised from taxes on petrol. The attention given to car driving as a major hazard to the public health can be judged by the fact that the World Health Organisation document on Health

Promotion devotes 12 lines to it (WHO, 1982). These concentrate solely on alcohol, drugs and seat-belt use. This comparative lack of interest not only creates the impression that hazards associated with motor cars are trivial relative to, say, lack of exercise, but simultaneously conveys the idea that it is a few irresponsible 'maniacs' who tank up themselves as well as their vehicles, drive carelessly and refuse to wear seat belts who are to blame for any hazards associated with cars. Thus attention is diverted from the enormous impact of car use on disease, death, disability, quality of life, the integrity of the environment, social intercourse, social inequalities and from the huge financial cost to the public purse.

Every private car should carry a government health warning.

Car driving kills or maims over 40,000 people every year in Britain

In 1982, there were 71,586 fatal or serious road accidents in Great Britain, the vast majority of which involved private cars. Of the surviving victims over half will have some permanent disability or disfigurement. The dictionary definition of accidental is 'occurring by chance; unexpected or unintentional; non-essential; incidental; without apparent cause'. In all these senses, except perhaps unintentional, the major proportion of incidents on the road are not accidents at all, but the foreseeable outcome of a combination of speed, carelessness, insensitivity, poor judgement, aggressive behaviour and egocentricity, sometimes aggravated by alcohol.

Although road accidents come fourth in the list of major causes of death, after lung, colon and breast cancer, they approximate lung cancer as the primary cause of years of life expectancy lost (Thunhurst, 1983). The peak years for the diagnosis of lung cancer are between ages 64 and 75, for coronary heart disease it is 55 to 64 years and for stroke it is over 75. By contrast, motor vehicle accidents are commonest in the under 40s and as a cause of death in children they approximate that of malignant neoplasms. In the City of Manchester, between 1980–1984, 35 per cent of all pedestrians and 28 per cent of all cyclists killed or seriously injured were children (Manchester City Council, 1986). In Britain, as a whole, pedestrian child fatalities in the age group 10–14 years has increased by 38 per cent in the last 10 years (TRRL, 1986).

About 16 people die every day on British roads, the same number as were shot on one occasion by Michael Ryan in an incident which led to the banning of certain types of weapons. Douglas Hurd, the Home Secretary, said that 'there can be no justification for a private individual wanting to hold a license for such a weapon'.

Now substitute 'vehicle' for 'weapon' and try applying another of the Home Secretary's remarks on this tragic event to private cars: 'Exceptionally good grounds will have to exist for their purchase and continued possession'.

In total there are about one and a half million *reported* 'accidents' on the roads every year in Britain, and last year there were about 12 million world-wide. The number of deaths resulting from these 'accidents', at around 6,000, is undoubtedly an underestimate, since deaths from, say, heart attack, which may have been triggered by the event are not included in the statistics. Moreover, injuries and conditions which are a consequence of road accidents and which result in death more than 30 days later are also not recorded as due to a road accident. Although the vast majority of 'accidents' involve private cars, half the people who die as a consequence are either pedestrians or cyclists (Hamer, 1985).

Most accidents to children occur in deprived urban areas where there is little play space. Boys in Social Class V are seven times more likely to be in an accident than those in Social Class I. Interestingly enough, the responsibility for this has usually been placed upon the child or upon his mother. The former for lack of road sense, impulsive behaviour or carelessness and the latter for lack of control or stress (Brown and Harris, 1978). Thus ameliorative measures have focused upon safety education for the children, or counselling and parental education for the mothers; a wonderful example of those who 'own' a problem trying to place responsibility for it onto less powerful groups, getting them to acknowledge the problem as belonging to them and urging them to change *their* behaviour accordingly (Gusfield, 1975).

Recent studies have shown that, in fact, children spend relatively small amounts of time in impulsive activities such as ball games; rather, for most of the time, they simply stand around or walk about (Chapman *et al.*, 1980). The association between stress in mothers and road accidents involving their children is probably an artefact of living in disadvantaged circumstances. Children from the lower social classes are less likely to have gardens or other play space and, therefore, spend more time in the streets. The real vulnerability of the children stems from their frequent daily exposure to risky situations, not their behaviour (Chapman *et al.*, 1980). Cars and other vehicles are allowed to pass through crowded urban streets which may even be widened and have obstacles removed to ensure traffic flow, leading to increased speed. Nicholas Ridley said in 1986, 'The motorist should not be hampered by petty rules and unnecessary restrictions of his liberty'. Is it an 'unnecessary restriction of liberty' to require that motorists drive slowly in urban areas if this will save the lives of several hundred children every year?

Studies of driving in urban areas have shown that no allowances are made by drivers for the presence of a child at the kerb (Chapman *et al.*, 1980). Most motorists maintain or increase speed, rarely do they slow down or move over to the crown of the road in anticipation. The 'jumping' of designated pedestrian crossing areas is not uncommon. Many drivers seem to assume that a car has the right to unimpeded progress.

It has been suggested, ironically enough, that measures pertaining to driver safety, for example seat-belts, padded fascia, better braking, improved acceleration, have resulted in increased accidents to other road users. Protecting car drivers from the consequences of their own follies can encourage careless driving and certainly faster driving (Adams, 1984).

Death is, of course, not necessarily the worst that can happen; injuries are more frequent and infinitely more distressing to the recipient. Front-seat passengers, who are more likely to be women than men, are injured more often and more severely than drivers. The consequences of this 'passive driving' are likely to be lacerations to the face. About 8 per cent of people involved in road accidents end up with permanent disabilities, including brain damage. World-wide, this means about one and a half million individuals, who, since they are mainly young, constitute a long-term drain on the energy, emotions and resources of their loved ones as well as on health and social services.

In spite of the very real dangers, however, few road users with the possible exception of cyclists, regard themselves, in the terms of Wordsworth, as 'travellers betwixt life and death'. The personal and financial cost has little impact on professionals or the lay public and most people are more afraid of flying even though it is much safer than car travel.

Public health economists have paid little attention to cost factors associated with motor vehicle accidents. In Scotland the estimated cost of *one* fatal accident is over £160,000 and last year the cost of all road accidents was in excess of £200 million. In Great Britain the total cost was £2,370 million (Plowden and Hillman, 1984).

Measures taken to reduce the burden of road accidents have generally focused on the convenience of the motorist and are designed to cause maximum inconvenience to others. Feeble old ladies and women with prams must struggle up steps and over bridges or scurry through stinking underpasses. Children unlucky enough to have no garden must confine themselves to the indoors or play at their peril. All such measures ignore the evidence that the main aetiological factor in deaths and injuries from road accidents is car driving itself.

Driving can damage your health and your environment

In towns and cities the foul and pestilent congregation of vapours which make up what is known as 'air' contains a large measure of car exhaust emissions. The most abundant of these is carbon monoxide, which is released in highly localised concentrations, especially in urban areas. High levels of this gas can hang in the air for extended periods of time. Levels as high as 100 parts per million (ppm) have been recorded at rush hours, reaching 350 ppm at peak times (Walker, 1975). These levels are sufficient to cause headache, lassitude and dizziness in normal people, since carbon monoxide interferes with the ability of the blood to carry oxygen due to its combination with haemoglobin. For susceptible people, for example, those who suffer from anaemia, have low haemoglobin levels, smokers and cardiovascular patients, the effects may be serious. Carbon monoxide at commonly occurring levels has been linked to aggravation of angina pectoris, atherosclerosis and stroke and has been implicated in poor survival rates from myocardial infarction (Goldsmith and Aronow, 1975).

Internal combustion also results in elevated levels of hydrocarbons. Photochemical oxidation creates derivatives from hydrocarbons which become secondary pollutants producing photochemical smog composed of ozone and other toxins. These cause eye irritation and plant damage, but the main problem is that they augment the effects of sulphur dioxide and nitrogen oxides (Duffus, 1980). Sulphur oxides are produced in comparatively small amounts by the combustion of fuel oil but the amount produced by cars adds to the output from industry and is a major cause of 'acid rain' through the oxidation of sulphates. Respiratory problems and eye irritation can be triggered by the inhalation of sulphur oxides at concentrations as low as 1.6 ppm. When concentrations of 5 ppm lasting for one hour occur, serious problems with respiration can ensue. Sulphate concentrations as low as two parts per billion have been found to adversely affect people with chronic respiratory problems, including asthmatics. This concentration is often exceeded in urban areas (Walker, 1975). Ironically, the introduction of catalytic units into cars, in an attempt to control CO and hydrocarbons, also results in an increase in the emission of sulphates.

Nitrogen oxides occur as nitric oxide and nitrogen dioxide. While nitric oxide mainly affects plants by interfering with photosynthesis, nitrogen dioxide penetrates mucus membranes and can affect breathing especially in susceptible people. Nitrogen emissions also contribute to the acidification of soil and water and the eutrophication of water, a process whereby over-enrichment of the water with nitrogen leads to excessive proliferation of small plants which, upon decomposition, deoxygenate the water, thus ensuring that other organisms will not survive (Duffus, 1980).

Recent attempts to eliminate lead from petrol in Britain have been delayed by the government, under pressure, no doubt, from powerful lobbies. Currently, there is about 400 mg of inorganic tetraethyl lead in every litre of petrol which, upon combustion, sticks to dust. Lead dust is washed by rain into drains or sewers contaminating water supplies and agricultural land, resulting in irreversible and cumulative poisoning of the earth. Organic lead is more toxic and can enter the body in a vapourous form. The maximum safe level is thought to be 35 micrograms per 100 millilitres of blood. However, one study of pre-school children in Birmingham found blood levels as high as 89 μg. Those children living in urban areas often have blood lead levels as high as 50–100 μg. Lead has been linked to still births, learning disorders and cognitive impairment, (Walker, 1981; Pihl and Parkes, 1977). Children are most at risk because they absorb up to 50 per cent of the lead in the food they consume whereas adults take in only 5–10 per cent. A recent study in Edinburgh by Fulton et al. (1987) found that blood lead levels were significantly associated with children's scores on reading, attainment and ability tests, when 33 possible confounding variables had been taken into account.

The lead content in British food is so high as to contravene international regulations largely as a consequence of vehicle emissions. It has been estimated that, for those vegetables with a high surface area, such as lettuce and broccoli there are few places where the crops are fit for consumption by infant humans (Russell Jones, 1981).

Diesel fuel may be even more harmful, in so far as thousands of chemicals, many of which are carcinogenic are breathed in from diesel fumes, exposure to which over a prolonged period results in a 42 per cent greater chance of developing lung cancer. It is predicted that diesel car ownership will grow in Europe from 5.8 million in 1986 to 15.5 million by 1995.

Many of the substances created by the internal combustion engine have a synergistic effect, so that whilst the impact of any single chemical may be relatively small, combinations of two or more, may have serious implications. There has been a growth of interest in vehicle emissions as a cause of lung, and possibly other, cancers. Robinson (1979) plotted the increase in cases of lung cancer in Australia between 1920 and 1972. Overall the percentage increase was 2,810 per cent. During the same period the increase in motor car use was 2,840 per cent, whilst tobacco use, for example, rose by only 69 per cent.

There is also some evidence that those who service and maintain cars such as garage hands, may be at risk from a variety of cancers (Theml, 1986). Although petrol engines have become cleaner over the years and total emissions are less, the increase in sheer volume of traffic has offset this and car use now accounts for a greater percentage of air and land pollution than it did 20 years ago (Ryan, 1980).

In addition to the health hazards associated with emissions, driving itself may have physical and emotional costs. For example, tachycardia is common when driving and the subsequent release of catecholamines is not dissipated in physical activity. The emotional reactions and task performance of car drivers have been found to be adversely affected for a time up to 2 hours after arrival at their destination. It appears that even routine experience of traffic congestion creates prolonged physiological arousal and an increase in blood pressure. Long-distance car commuters have been found to have a higher incidence of coronary heart disease, ulcers and stomach disorders than a matched group of short distance commuters (Stokols *et al.*, 1978). Driving is also known to be a common factor provoking angina pectoris (Taggart *et al.*, 1969). An unknown percentage of 'accidents' are a consequence of drivers having heart attacks at the wheel. A recent *Guardian* report, for example, described the death of a 25-year-old mother and her 3-year-old twins when they were hit by a car after the driver suffered a fatal heart attack. This may be regarded as no more a 'chance' occurrence than selling a hand gun to a man with a history of violence.

Comparative controlled studies of the health effects of driving itself are quite rare and there is a need for more work in this area. Car driving is now one of the commonest activities in the Western world. A great many people spend many hours engaged in it or, in the case of traffic jams, being frustrated by not being able to engage in it.

A further health hazard stems from the noise levels generated by road traffic, which is the major contributor to total noise levels in the UK creating a background of intermittent noise which is augmented by revving engines, slamming doors and blaring radios. Approximately one-third of the population live in areas where noise levels are high enough to cause health problems. Continual exposure to traffic noise has been found to increase heart rate, blood pressure and adrenalin output, which if added to other strains may culminate in chronic hypertension and damage to heart function (Andren, 1982; Ising et al., 1980). In addition, uncontrollable and unpredictable noise has a clear stressing effect, especially when it is intermittent (A.A.S., 1976). Decreases in work performance are associated with traffic noise and there is some evidence that it accentuates failing hearing with age (Rossi, 1976). The general arousal effect of noise associated with traffic disturbs sleep patterns and a study of motorway noise conducted in the homes of nearby residents showed that they took longer to fall asleep after the construction of the road; had, on average, 16 minutes less deep sleep than formerly and showed a reduction in REM sleep. There was no adaptation to the noise 5 years later. Sleep disturbances such as these are known to have adverse psychological and physiological consequences (Gloag, 1980).

There are other indirect health effects of car use. At a time when the populace are being urged to take more exercise, the cheapest and possibly best forms of activity, walking and cycling are discouraged by motor traffic. Surveys have indicated that many more people would walk to work, to the shops and for leisure, if the roads were less noisy, dirty and dangerous (Morton, Williams et al., 1978). In addition, the perception of danger effectively distorts the travel of others by deterring their own excursions. The elderly and disabled may prefer not to go out at all rather than cope with the roads. Likewise an old person or a child may require someone to accompany them to ensure their safety.

A study by Waldman (1977) found that the main deterrents to cycling were hills, danger from traffic and rain. The expected level of cycling in a flat but dangerous town was 6 per cent of all traffic, while in a safe town it was 43 per cent of traffic. This has been confirmed by studies in Holland (Dutch National Survey, 1978). When facilities are provided huge increases of 40 per cent and more occur in the use of bicycles for journeys to school, work and the shops (Kolks, 1981). In Sweden and Japan where car use has been discouraged in favour of other means of transport, especially cycling, there has been a 25 per cent decrease in accidents to cyclists and a 31 per cent decrease in accidents to pedestrians, in addition to substantial reductions in noise and pollution. Cycle use, as well as being a source of exercise and enjoyment, requires only 7 per cent of the total energy required by a car, including fuel, repairs, maintenance and production. The increase in car ownership over the last few decades appears to have influenced exercise levels. Since there has been very little change in per capita energy consumption over this time it is tempting to speculate that car ownership has played a part in the increase in the number of people who are overweight. We have now reached a ludicrous situation where physical exercise requires special provision, jogging suits, time set aside and designated sports areas instead of being built into the flow of daily activity. People may drive 3 miles to work and then have to use the time they 'saved' taking exercise.

A spokesman for the British Motor Industry Heritage Trust, not perhaps without his own biases, recently opined that, 'Freedom of mobility is as great a freedom as that of speech or political independence and a private motor car offers that mobility'. Let us suppose that the motorist is able to escape the motorway crawl and the urban traffic jam and reach what is left of the countryside, or the coast, what is likely to be found there? Most often there will be a lot of other motor cars, some ugly parking areas, litter, perhaps a few derelict cars which can be glimpsed scattered down a hillside. Easier access for cars creates more congestion, tiny villages become impassable, the shoreline and the countryside become parking lots. In the interest of traffic flow there will have been planned and systematic removal of aesthetically important features of towns and villages. Agricultural land is encroached upon, beauty desecrated, ugliness created and plants and animals disturbed, if not destroyed entirely. The private car progressively destroys amenities at the same time as it ensures less mobility for walkers and cyclists.

Car driving can ruin your character

It is a popular prejudice that people change when they get behind the wheel. Whether they change or just display characteristics usually submerged in the normative niceties of social intercourse, the behaviour of many drivers, whether deliberate or not, displays an anarchic, aggressive and anti-social tendency which would earn them ostracism if not a thick ear when on foot. It seems likely that some of these tendencies are encouraged by a degree of sensory and social isolation giving the illusion of separation from a social context such that the usual obligations and empathies of everyday life are suspended.

Imagine, for example, a pedestrian behaving in the following manner:

> Getting close behind another pedestrian and maintaining the same speed meanwhile flashing a torch at them.
>
> On being overtaken by another pedestrian, speeding up and then immediately pulling up in front of her.
>
> On rainy days throwing large quantities of water over people standing at the kerbside.
>
> If about to be passed by another pedestrian speeding up – whereupon the other will also speed up and so on, until both are proceeding along the High Street at break-neck speed, endangering other pedestrians.
>
> Walking along the street making obscene gestures, swearing at other pedestrians merely for being there and criticising the way they walk.

If these behaviours were indulged in by pedestrians they might easily be regarded as evidence of severe mental disorder.

A car appears to engender a feeling of privacy, even though it is in the public domain, and a feeling of urgency, even though none exists. The speed limit is now routinely broken and the Highway Code is often disregarded. Although a pedestrian has right of way when crossing a side street, few car drivers acknowledge this and are much more likely to speed round the corner sounding their horn in the expectation that the pedestrian will give way which, unless the person is suicidal, will invariably happen.

Certain aspects of irresponsibility in motorists are officially encouraged. A driver who has been drinking and subsequently kills someone can be and often is accused of careless driving, fined a paltry sum or receives an endorsement on their licence, in spite of the fact that the decision to take alcohol and then take charge of a lethal weapon, must be regarded as criminal in moral, if not legal, terms. The number of convictions for drunken driving rose from 58,000 in 1976 to 107,000 in 1986, probably as a result of breath-testing. Whatever the reason, it is clear that a large number of potential killers are released on to our roads every day, their judgment seriously impaired. Speeding is now so commonplace that the police often do not bother to prosecute unless the speed attained is very high, say over 100 m.p.h. Even so the penalties incurred are quite small.

Private cars or public transport?

Public transport, especially in Britain, has, in the past few years, been dramatically reduced, whilst road-building to cope with car traffic has proceeded at unprecedented rates.

As well as being convenient, bus travel is safer than any other form of transport. Low bus fares led to a decline in accident rates in the London area in 1981, rates which increased at an estimated cost of £20 million when fares were increased in 1982 (Controller of Transport and Development, 1983). A study by Nicholl *et al.* (1987) of the effects of bus subsidies in South Yorkshire between 1975 and 1986 showed that bus travel increased there relative to other metropolitan counties and that, since buses are the safest form of travel, the health of the local population benefited. In addition, buses are more energy efficient and take up an infinitesimal amount of space per passenger mile as compared to a car.

Rail travel is also relatively safe and allows travelling time to be used for other pursuits, such as reading, working, playing games or drinking beer. Motor cars are extremely inefficient in energy terms, because they are designed for speeds in excess of 80 m.p.h. which are rarely attained. They are, according to Mumford (1954), little better than the first steam engine which wasted most of its energy in radiation and noise. Before the advent of the private car, approximately 50,000 people crossed London Bridge on foot every hour. Cars can move, at most, 24,000 people, often less, in the same period of time. In terms of space, a car takes up 80 square feet for every 1.4 persons, while a bus can carry 33 occupants for the same amount of room.

Unfortunately, a vicious cycle has arisen whereby the decline in the availability of public transport has led to an increase in the use of the private car, thus justifying the decline in public transport at severe inconvenience to poorer rural and urban dwellers, the elderly, women and children, whose freedom of mobility is increasingly curtailed. Recent reports have highlighted the extent to which women in particular are discriminated against in transport policy. In the last ten years spending on road construction and maintenance has risen by 30 per cent. However, only one-third of women possess a driving licence and far fewer have access to a car on a daily basis. Schemes that are designed to speed up and facilitate traffic flow hinder the mobility of women by reducing or slowing down public transport or forcing them, literally, underground. The location of supermarkets, hospitals, schools and clinics, where women form a majority of visitors may require a long and involved trip by bus, as opposed to a short and simple journey by car (London Strategic Policy Unit, 1988; Transport 2000, 1988). Incidentally, one little remarked upon effect of the building of peripheral supermarkets is an increase in the prices in local shops whose share of the available trade is inevitably diminished. Once again the poor, the elderly, the disabled and the non-motorist are penalised and social inequalities are exacerbated.

The sheer amount of space given over to cars and other vehicles is quite remarkable. Not only do cars occupy a disproportionate amount of the ground area available but they also routinely encroach on to pedestrian areas, pavements and grassy places. Thus pedestrians are faced with having to squeeze past vehicles on the pavement, sometimes being forced into the roadway themselves. Signs for motorists are invariably sited on pedestrian space – the pavement. Needless to say, this is not a reciprocal arrangement.

Conclusions

The daily confrontations between frail flesh and lethal metal have come to seem normal. The dominance of the car in the landscape, the spoilation of towns, villages and countryside continues to go almost unquestioned, except by a few cranks. Most individuals assume that they have an automatic right to possess a weapon which kills and maims many more people every year than do rifles or guns. Far from being regarded as anti-social, the private car has been elevated to a status symbol, a cause for pride, a target of devotion. Even people who are aware of the problems associated with car ownership will plead that a car is a necessity rather as others might argue that they need a cigarette or a drink to help them cope with the exigencies of daily life.

The encouragement of car ownership is just as much a product of powerful lobbies as is smoking or alcohol use. Industrial societies subsidise motorists to a large extent (Bouladon, 1975). The car and oil industry, motoring organisations and road contractors exert their influence in the interests of private profit at enormous cost to the public purse. The drain on the public sector is not due solely to the cost of accidents and disability, hours lost at work or health services provided, but includes noise, vibration, congestion, damage to buildings, loss of time, waste of space, high energy consumption, pollution and inconvenience to others, especially those already at a disadvantage by virtue of age, sex or infirmity. In addition to the cost of 'accidents', congestion alone is estimated to cost the country £3,000 million in lost time and wasted fuel (GMCP, 1987).

The risks to life, limb and environment associated with cars are either ignored or treated as an acceptable price to pay (acceptable to motorists that is). Yet the number of people who will be killed on the roads between now and 1990 will far exceed the projected number of AIDS victims, and the number of people disabled for life will be many times greater; yet the resources and time devoted to this serious public health problem are far, far fewer. We have reached the ludicrous situation in Britain where the success of transport policy is measured by the number of vehicles that can travel at high speed to the detriment of everything else, a criterion comparable to measuring the success of health policy by the number of people who pass through hospitals.

Smoking, alcohol and drug use, dietary habits and lack of exercise are constantly targeted as 'unhealthy' and responsible for major diseases and disabilities, in spite of only meagre supporting evidence. Car use, on the other hand, is indisputably 'unhealthy' in a variety of ways, but as a 'risk factor' it is rarely cited. The perception and selection of risks is not independent of selectors. Cars are an unpopular target for the new public health reformers because they themselves are often car owners. The middle classes are less likely to smoke, but regard a car, even two, as essential.

If there is a recognition of risk, it is assumed that a combination of road and car design coupled with driver education will minimise the danger. However, the first merely transfers the problem to put other members of the public at risk and the second is as naïve a concept as health education in relation to, say, exercise, since it ignores the social context within which car driving is seen as a desirable behaviour and the complex pressure from interested parties.

Some countries are making efforts to assign a more subordinate role to the private car. In the Netherlands and Scandinavia, very low speeds are enforced in urban areas by environmental design and pedestrians, cyclists and the landscape are assigned higher priority than vehicular traffic. One result of this is the lowest pedestrian accident rates in Europe; less than half that in Britain where the opposite strategy seems to prevail. In Scotland, for example, although The Roads (Scotland) Act (1984) allows for the construction of road bumps to slow down traffic (well done Scotland!), the former Minister for Home Affairs and the Environment, Michael Ancram, refused to commit himself to the introduction of road bumps on the grounds that they were 'potential dangers' and that the 'interests of road safety must be paramount' (Ancram, 1985). There can be no doubt that it is the motorist who is of major concern here and not the potential victims.

The traditional way of dealing with car accidents has been to try to contain the number and severity in relation to a given volume of traffic (Plowden and Hillman, 1984). It would, however, make more sense to encourage alternative means of travel and, by creating more public awareness of the totality of hazards associated with private cars, encourage a demand for a more comprehensive and responsive public transport system.

Although most drivers justify the use of cars in terms of convenience and time saved it is doubtful whether this could be justified empirically. Most time in a car is spent waiting with the engine running, a state which is the most wasteful of energy and also the most polluting. If looking after the car, washing it, parking it, getting fuel, finding where it is parked, getting it repaired, sitting or crawling in traffic and doing associated paper work, were taken into account and totalled over a week or a year, car ownership would be likely to constitute a much greater expenditure of time and resources than a bicycle or even public transport plus walking.

All forms of public transport, buses and trains, monorails and subway systems are cheaper, safer and more energy efficient than the private car per passenger mile. Even taxis are less costly for the passenger than the price, upkeep and running of a private car, which is often not in use for most of the time. Taxis which carry a number of people not necessarily sharing the same destination as, for example, the Israeli Sherut, are clearly much less wasteful.

Walking and cycling would undoubtedly increase if they could be carried out in safety and pleasant surroundings. Local authorities could do much here to support cycle paths and discourage road building and urban throughways. It is vehicles which should be required to use underpasses and bridges not pedestrians. Anyone who is concerned about loss of life, disfigurement and disability, environmental pollution and social inequalities can make a statement by relinquishing his or her car, lobbying Members of Parliament and local councillors, refusing to use peripheral supermarkets and discouraging car use by others. Controls on car advertisements, comparable to those on cigarette advertising, should be introduced, whereby promotional material likely to encourage excessive speed would be banned. All motoring offences need to be treated with more seriousness – not solely those committed by people with excess alcohol in their blood. Irresponsibility is not confined to those who drink and drive or who ignore speed limits and safety advice, it extends to everyone who contributes to the serious public health problems caused by private cars.

References

Adams, J. (1984) *Sneed's law, seat belts and the empower's new clothes*, London: Department of Geography, University College.

Ancram, M. (1985) Letter to Michael Hurst, M.P. (personal communication from K. Sutherland).

Andren, L. (1982) Cardiovascular effects of noise, *Acta Med Scand*, Suppl. 657, 1–45.

Australian Academy of Science (1976) Report of a Committee on the Problem of Noise, Canberra: Report No. 20.

Bouladon, G. (1979) Costs and benefits of motor vehicles, in *Urban Transport and the Environment*, Paris: O.E.C.D., 277–319.

Brown, G. and Harris, T. (1978) *Social Origins of Depression, a Study of Psychiatric Disorder in Women*, London: Tavistock.

Chapman, A. J., Foot, H. and Wade, F. (1980) Children at play, in D. J. Osborne and J. A. Levis (eds) *Human Factors in Transport Research* vol. 2, London: Academic Press.

Controller of Transport and Development (1983) Report to the Transport Commission of the Greater London Council. Hem T937, London, October.

Dutch National Travel Survey (1978), The Hague.

Fulton, M., Thomson, G., Hunter, R. *et al.* (1987) Influence of blood lead on the ability and attainment of children in Edinburgh, *Lancet*, May 30th, 1221–6.

Gloag, D. (1980) Noise and health: public and private responsibility, *British Medical Journal*, *281*, 1404–7.

Greater Manchester Cycling Project (1987) Stop the Child Slaughter, G.M.C.P., Occasional Paper No. 2, August, Manchester.

Cusfield, J. (1975) Categories of ownership and responsibility in social issues: alcohol abuse and automobile use, *Journal of Drug Issues, 5*, 290–5.

Hamer, M. (1985) How speed kills on Britain's roads, *New Scientist*, 21st February, 10–11.

Hartunian, N. S., Smart C. N. and Thompson, M. S. (1980) The incidence and economic costs of cancer, motor vehicle incidents, coronary heart disease and stroke: a comparative analysis, *American Journal of Public Health*, *70*, 1249–60.

Ising, H. Dienel, D. Gunther, T. and Markert, B. (1980) Health effects of traffic noise, *Int. Arch. Occup. Env. Hlth*, *47*, 179–90.

Kilks, A. (1981) Bocholt – a town for cyclists, in *Proceedings of the 1st International Bicycle Congress VELO/CITY*, Bremen: West Germany Federal Ministry of Transport, April.

Kitsuse, J. and Spector, M. (1975) Social problems and deviance: some parallel issues, *Social Problems*, *36*, 584–94.

London Strategic Policy Unit (1988) *Women's safe transport in London*, London: LSPU.

Manchester City Council (1986) *Interim Report of the Black Report Working Party on Accidents to Children, Manchester.*

Morton-Williams, T., Hedges, B. and Fernando, E. (1978) *Road Traffic and the Environment*, London: Social and Community Planning Research.

Mumford, L. (1954) In defence of neighbourhood, *Town Planning Review*, 24, 256–70.

Nicholl, J. P., Freeman, M. R. and Williams, B. T. (1987) Effects of subsidising bus travel on the occurrence of road traffic casualties, *Journal of Epidemiology and Community Health*, 41, 50–4.

Pihl, R., and Parkes, M. (1977) Hair element content in learning disabled children, *Science*, 204–09.

Plowden, S. and Hillman, M. (1984) *Danger on the Road: The Needless Scourge*, London: Policy Studies Institute.

Robinson, A. A. (1979) Does driving cause cancer and diabetes?, *Medical Hypotheses*, 5, 175–184.

Rossi, G. (1976) Urban traffic noise: auditory and extra auditory effects, *Acta Oto-Laryncology*, Suppl., 339.

Russell Jones, R. (1981) Lead poisoning: why the government must act now, *World Medicine*, February, 73.

Ryan, G. A. (1980) The automobile and human health, in N. F. Stanley and R. A. Joske (eds) *Changing Disease Patterns and Human Behaviour*, London: Academic Press, 468–90.

Stokols, D., Novaco, R. W., Stokols, J. and Campbell, J. (1978) Traffic congestion, Type A behaviour and stress, *Journal of Applied Psychology*, 63, 467–80.

Taggart, P., Gibbons, D. and Somerville, W. (1969) Some effects of motor car driving on the normal and abnormal heart, *British Medical Journal*, iv, 130–4.

Theml, H. (1986) Um Leib und Leben: medizinische Auswirkungen des Auto verkehrs, in P. M. Bode, Sylvia Hemberger, W. Zangl et al. (eds) *Alptraum Auto*, Hamburg: Raben Verlag.

Thunhurst, C. (1983) Fares fair – the health case for cheap fares, *Radical Community Medicine*, 15, Autumn, 1–7.

Transport and Road Research Laboratory (1986) Press Notice No. 6, 28th October.

Transport 2000, London.

Waldman, J. (1977) *Cycling in towns: a quantitative investigation*, LTRI Working Paper No. 3, London: Department of Transport.

Walker, H. (1981) Is lead the key to perinatal mortality? *World Medicine*, August, 20.

World Health Organisation (1982) *Lifestyles Conducive to Health. Regional Strategy for attaining HFA by year 2000*, Copenhagen: WHO, Regional Office for Europe.

10

PAMELA GILLIES

HEALTH BEHAVIOUR AND HEALTH PROMOTION IN YOUTH

Introduction

Recent evidence has revealed that health behaviours in youth such as smoking and drinking remain a significant potential source of future health problems in young people in the UK. Among 15–16-year-olds approximately one in five boys (19 per cent) and one in three girls (30 per cent) are smoking regularly (OPCS, 1987). Half of the 17-year-olds in England and Wales report drinking at least weekly and, although most teenagers report modest levels of consumption, three-quarters of Scottish 17-year-old boys consume upwards of five pints of beer on a Saturday night (OPCS, 1987). The prevention of unhealthy behaviours and maintenance of low-risk activity must therefore remain a priority for health promotion in youth.

Health promotion and educational programmes for youth have been informed by research which has identified factors associated with smoking and drinking in children and adolescents. The vast majority of the UK findings to date have, however, resulted from cross-sectional studies. Whilst such studies, particularly if repeated, can accurately determine important factors, they proffer little on patterns of initiation, maintenance, change in behaviours over time or factors associated with such changes, and whether such factors encourage smoking or drinking or are merely correlates.

Two major UK studies have adopted longitudinal cohort designs in an attempt to isolate predictive factors for smoking and drinking in teenagers. In a questionnaire study of 11-year-old children from

116

1974–78, Murray *et al.* (1983) found that the significant factors which predicted smoking included: parental or sibling smoking; having friends of the opposite sex; participation in social activities such as discos or cinema; non-participation in sporting activities; and, in girls, dissatisfaction with school. Murray *et al.* concluded that attention should be paid to the changing social context in which teenagers develop the smoking habit, if the uptake and maintenance of the habit at different stages in adolescence is to be explained further.

Many studies of alcohol use in youth have concentrated upon the antecedents or factors associated with problem drinking (Fillmore, 1974; Donovan *et al.*, 1983). However, in a longitudinal study of alcohol, tobacco and drug misuse, Plant *et al.* (1985) did note that smoking at the age of 15 was a predictive factor for alcohol consumption 4 years later. Plant *et al.* also found that alcohol was usually used in the company of friends, particularly whilst at discos, and that alcohol misuse at the age of 15 predicted the use of illicit drugs but did not predict alcohol consumption 4 years later. In both studies, the authors pointed to the 'social' nature of smoking or drinking in youth.

The preliminary findings of the longitudinal study reported here identified predictive factors for a series of healthy and potentially unhealthy behaviours in youth by using a more broadly based approach than previously. The collection of quantitative data using an open- as well as a closed-question format was complemented by qualitative information. The interview aimed to: explore adolescents' reasons for their health related behaviour choices; how such reasons changed as teenagers matured; and locate behaviours within the social context in which they occurred.

Methods

Sample. In 1984 a sample of 1,797 teenagers aged 11–16 years from fourteen randomly selected schools in Nottingham completed a questionnaire. This paper describes a sub-set of the findings for those 584 pupils who were 11 years old in March 1984. In March 1987, 503 of these pupils were successfully followed up when aged 14 years (86 per cent response rate) and completed the same questionnaire a second time. In addition, it is intended to interview all of these 503 pupils and, to date, 152 interviews (77 boys; 75 girls) have been completed and are described here. Data were linked longitudinally by birth data recorded in the questionnaire.

Data collection. Data were collected using a self-completed confidential questionnaire administered by classroom teachers, a

Table 10.1. Significant risk factors for weekly drinking at 11 and 14 years

Factor	Drink weekly N	%	Don't drink weekly N	%	Age	Relative odds (drinking to not drinking weekly)	Confidence limits	X^2	Significance
Male—Yes	76	26	234	74	11	1.76	1.16–2.67	6.44	$p<0.02$
No	41	16	222	84					
Male—Yes	93	38	151	62	14	1.36	1.16–1.95	4.99	$p<0.05$
No	70	28	178	72					
Ever smoking	49	26	59	17	11	1.88	1.23–2.89	7.79	$p<0.01$
Regular smoking	30	56	127	31	14	2.54	1.46–4.42	10.01	$p<0.01$
Intend to smoke	21	40	95	18	11	2.99	1.68–5.32	12.65	$p<0.001$
	28	56	134	31	14	2.89	1.62–5.13	11.94	$p<0.001$
Best friend smokes	23	32	67	18	11	2.17	1.25–3.77	6.72	$p<0.01$
Dislike school	30	29	45	17	11	1.98	1.17–3.35	5.78	$p<0.02$
Disco once a week	102	41	56	25	14	2.08	1.41–3.08	12.80	$p<0.001$
Social class I or II	33	48	101	33	14	1.61	0.90–2.83	8.47	$p<0.02$

procedure which is known, in the case of smoking, to produce the highest rates of self-reported smoking (McKennal, 1980). The questionnaire covered many aspects of health-related behaviour including smoking, drinking, diet, exercise, sleep, self-medication, in a series of closed questions. This paper concentrates upon smoking and alcohol consumption. Thoughts, hopes for and worries about the future were recorded in open questions. Data on social class were compiled from adolescents' self-reports of their father's occupation, and comparison of self-reported data with available census data for Nottingham on social class reveals a marked similarity.

The validity of self-reported data on smoking (Evans *et al.*, 1980) and drinking (Midaink, 1982) has been challenged on the grounds that young people are likely to either under-report because they perceive it to be socially unacceptable to indulge in the behaviour or alternatively over-report to boast. However, evidence does exist to suggest that adolescents do provide accurate reports of their smoking (Gillies, 1985; Williams and Gillies, 1985) and drinking behaviour (Plant *et al.*, 1985).

Additional information was gained by structured interviews lasting upwards of 30 minutes. All interviews were carried out by one female researcher, in a room in the school set aside for that purpose. Boys and girls were equally co-operative at interview.

Results

The significant risk factors for smoking and drinking in youth are compared and any changes between the age of 11 and 14 years identified.

Drinking. As Table 10.1 shows, at the age of 11 and 14 years, weekly drinkers were more likely to be male than female, to have smoked, and to say they intend to smoke in the future. At the age of 11, weekly drinkers may be drinking and smoking with their friends whilst expressing their 'dislike' of school. At the age of 14, weekly drinkers were, in addition to being more likely to smoke, also more likely to engage in mixed sex activities such as going to discos. The findings also suggest that 14-year-old drinkers may be more likely to be social class I or II. However, these latter data must be treated with caution due to the small number in this category and the fact that the lowest estimate of association given in the confidence limits suggests that there may be no relationship. In other words, this may be a chance finding, a suggestion underpinned by the fact that no other social class differences were recorded in relation to any other health behaviour related variable in this study.

Smoking. Smokers at 11 and 14 years of age were more likely

Table 10.2. Significant risk factors for smoking at 11 and 14 years

Factor	Smoke* N	Smoke* %	Don't smoke N	Don't smoke %	Age	Relative odds (smoking to non-smoking)	Confidence limits	X^2	Significance
Mother smokes	90	50	121	37	11	1.69	1.17–2.44	7.40	$p<0.01$
	34	63	147	37	14	2.87	1.62–5.08	12.04	$p<0.001$
Intends to smoke	29	16	16	5	11	3.79	2.07–6.93	17.22	$p<0.001$
	36	65	13	3	14	57.13	32.5–100.5	190.64	$p<0.001$
Best friend smokes	46	30	22	8	11	4.68	2.77–7.91	31.59	$p<0.001$
	45	85	51	14	14	35.63	19.5–65.1	131.24	$p<0.001$
Smoking helps you when you're nervous	82	58	75	35	11	2.55	1.66–3.93	17.23	$p<0.001$
	41	85	112	50	14	5.91	2.73–12.78	18.98	$p<0.001$
Drinks at least weekly	59	31	49	14	11	2.73	1.79–4.17	20.71	$p<0.001$
	30	54	127	31	14	2.54	1.46–4.42	10.01	$p<0.01$
Thinks health is middling to poor	39	21	46	13	11	1.69	1.06–2.69	4.34	$p<0.05$
	30	54	83	20	14	4.50	2.61–7.76	27.60	$p<0.001$
Dislikes school	51	40	48	21	11	2.60	1.63–4.16	14.99	$p<0.001$
	30	77	75	34	14	6.36	3.07–13.17	23.02	$p<0.001$

* Refers to ever-smoking in 11-year-olds and regular smokers ($\geqslant 1$ cigarette per week) in 14-year-olds.

to have mothers who smoke (especially girls), intend to smoke when older, have friends who smoke, think smoking helps when you're nervous, drink weekly, rarely exercise, dislike school and think their health is middling to poor as opposed to good to very good (Table 10.2). There were some differences by age. At 11 years smokers were more likely to be male; at the age of 14 years they are three times as likely to be female (6 per cent of boys compared with 18 per cent of girls). At 11 years they were more likely to go to discos and have friends who think it's 'cool' to smoke. Smoking therefore has strong associations with social activity in the younger adolescent, as does drinking weekly.

The older smoker, who is more likely to be female, was four times more likely than her non-smoking counterpart to be uncertain as to what the future holds for her in respect of a job or a place in college, and was twice as likely to feel low or irritable at least once a week (Table 10.3).

Worries for the future. The responses to the open questions on young peoples' hopes and fears for the future helped explain some of the risk factors for smoking at age 14 years. Large proportions of teenagers spontaneously expressed concern about unemployment, war, health matters, money, and AIDS. No social class differences in the extent or nature of worries were reported; therefore, like health behaviour, these concerns appear to cut across social class.

More youngsters reported worries with increasing age and at 14 years of age in interview, girls expressed more worries than boys, although it is difficult to determine whether this was due to girls really having more worries or to them expressing these more readily in interview than boys. However, of the 75 girls interviewed so far, 15 declared themselves to be smokers. Of this group, 12 indicated spontaneously that they used smoking as a coping strategy – to calm their nerves, help them get through the day and cope with all their worries. None of the males or females interviewed mentioned using alcohol in this way. It was used for a 'high', to change mood and be sociable. Drugs, soft or hard, were mentioned by only one of the young people interviewed.

Discussion

Many of the preliminary findings of this study concur with those of the two previous longitudinal investigations of drinking and smoking in youth.

As in the study by Plant *et al.* (1985), drinking was found to be strongly associated with smoking and with social activities with

Table 10.3. Significant risk factors for smoking at 11 and 14 years

Factor	Smoke* N	%	Don't smoke N	%	Age	Relative odds (smoking to non-smoking)	Confidence limits	X^2	Significance
Male—Yes	120	42	163	58	11	1.96	1.36–2.80	12.70	$p<0.001$
No	70	27	186	73					
Female—Yes	41	18	189	82	14	3.17	1.74–5.76	13.19	$p<0.001$
No	15	6	218	94					
Disco's at least weekly	105	58	143	43	11	1.82	1.27–2.62	9.86	$p<0.01$
Best friend thinks it's great you smoke	91	65	61	25	11	5.58	3.61–8.61	58.58	$p<0.001$
Uncertain what future holds (re jobs/school)	18	26	34	8	14	4.00	2.18–7.32	18.26	$p<0.001$
Feel 'low' at least once a week	20	36	79	20	14	2.29	1.27–4.11	6.68	$p<0.01$
Feel irritable or bad tempered at least once a week	35	63	149	37	14	2.84	1.62–4.98	12.30	$p<0.001$
Rarely sports or exercises outside school	22	43	81	21	14	2.93	1.63–5.27	11.70	$p<0.001$

friends of both sexes, such as going to discos. In 15-year-old adolescents Plant *et al.* also found a social class differential in alcohol use with highest use, in social class III and lowest in I and II. Given that the questions employed in this study were different and the age of students slightly younger (14 as opposed to 15 years and over), it is interesting to note that teenagers were more likely to drink weekly if they were social class I and II. The association was not strong, however, and the result may have been a chance finding, a suggestion underpinned by the fact that no other social class differences were recorded in relation to any other health behaviour related variable in this study. This latter finding parallels West's (1986) report on the absence of social class differences in mortality and morbidity in adolescence. If the association were 'real', it may perhaps be explained by accessibility to alcohol either due to pocket-money or due to access to well-stocked liquor cabinets in the home.

In relation to smoking, like Murray *et al.* (1983), this study found that parental smoking, especially in mothers, intention to smoke, dislike of school and non-participation in sporting activities were all significant predictors of smoking. However, whilst this study found that social activity, such as going to discos, strongly predicted smoking in the younger adolescent (11 years), a different picture emerged for the older adolescent (14 years) when the smoker was more likely to be female than male.

Risk factors for smoking in these older adolescents included the belief that smoking helped you when nervous, being uncertain as to what the future held and feeling 'low' at least once a week. These older adolescents, especially girls, reported at interview 'using' smoking to calm their nerves and cope with the large number of everyday worries they mentioned in open questions. These worries included unemployment, exams, concern about war, AIDs and their own health. The study did not assess the extent of worry, merely reported the numbers of worries expressed spontaneously. Therefore, whilst smoking and drinking are influenced by and maintained in adolescence through social activities in the main, there is a significant group of teenagers who are now using smoking as a coping strategy. These 'new' findings appear to be related to the increase in smoking in girls in recent years. The 1978 data reported by Murray *et al.* in 1983 recorded more adolescent boys than girls smoking. This situation has now been reversed.

The preliminary findings of this study may have the following implications for health education strategy to prevent smoking in youth:

Table 10.4. Adolescents' worries for the future (all choices combined)*

	11 years 1984		14 years 1987		Significance of difference between years
	N	%	N	%	
Unemployment	210	40	247	63	p<0.001
War	189	36	141	30	—
Own death	96	18	112	24	p<0.05
Money	98	18	113	24	p<0.05
AIDS	0	0	97	21	p<0.001
Poor health	88	17	58	12	—
Marriage	95	18	48	10	p<0.001
Childbirth	22	4	49	10	p<0.001
Exams	66	14	60	13	—
Parents death	60	11	45	10	—
Total sample	210		470		
Non-response	54		33		

* Respondents could give up to 3 worries.

Preventing the uptake of unhealthy behaviours. School education, using a combination of practical, science-based projects like the HEC My Body Project (HEC, 1983), discussion of peer-group and other influences on smoking (e.g. advertising) and the unsociable nature of the habit, have been shown substantially to reduce the risk of young people taking up smoking (Gillies and Wilcox, 1984).

The materials use young peoples' own language and use relevant examples. It remains to be seen whether the rates of smoking prevention achieved using these methods can be maintained beyond the age of 14 years. Such methods have recently also been applied to AIDS education (Gillies *et al.*, 1987) and alcohol education (Tacade, 1985) and should continue to be developed and implemented.

Developing coping mechanisms for youth. It follows that if a significant proportion of young people are smoking to cope with worries, then health education should be turning its attention to encouraging teenagers to deal with their anxieties by means other than smoking. New educational approaches need to be devised and tested.

Produce an enabling environment. If young people are encouraged to take responsibility for their own health and change their own behaviour, it is important that their efforts are set against the background of an environment which is reinforcing, at a local and national level. With respect to smoking, for example, the removal of cigarette advertising, which has now been shown to reinforce smoking in teenagers (Potts *et al.*, 1986), and the creation of no–smoking environments, would help establish an enabling environment.

Remove the root causes of young peoples' anxieties. It would be naïve to suggest that teenagers' worries about topics such as unemployment, AIDS and war can be relieved by action at governmental level. However, awareness of teenagers' concerns may be raised at local level, leading to local action. It may not be advisable to remove such concerns altogether, since apathy may result from stifling the 'voice' of young people.

These preliminary findings indicate that health promotion activities in youth must invoke both individual and community-based strategies. The current emphasis upon lifestyle and behaviour change in youth may only have a transient impact unless it is harnessed to social and physical changes in the environment.

References

Donovan, J. E., Jessor, R. and Jessor, L. (1983) Problem drinking in adolescence and young adulthood: a follow-up study, *Journal of Studies on Alcohol*, 44, 109–37.

Evans, R. T., Henderson, A. H., Hill, P. C. and Raines, B. E. (1979) Current psychological, social and educational programmes in the control and prevention of smoking: a critical methodological review, *Atherosclerosis Review*, 6, 204–43.

Fillmore, K. M. (1974) Drinking and problem drinking in early adulthood and middle age: an exploratory 20 year follow-up study, *Quarterly Journal of Studies on Alcohol*, 35, 819–40.

Gillies, P. A. and Wilcox, B. (1984) Reducing the risk of smoking amongst the young, *Public Health*, 98, 49–54.

Gillies, P. A. (1985) Accuracy in the measurement of smoking in young people, *Health Education Journal*, 44, 36–8.

Gillies, P. A., Roberts, H. and Bretman, M. (1987) *Young peoples' knowledge of AIDS and the need to get 'Streetwize'*, Department of Community Medicine and Epidemiology, University of Nottingham.

Health Education Council (1983) *My Body Project Materials*, London: Heinemann.

McKennel, A. C. (1980) Bias in the reported incidence of smoking by children, *International Journal of Epidemiology*, 9, 166–77.

Midaink, L. (1982) The validity of self-reported alcohol consumption and alcohol problems: a literature review, *British Journal of Addiction*, *77* (4), 357–82.

Murray, M., Swan, A. V., Bewley, B. R. and Johnson, M. R. D. (1983) The development of smoking during adolescence – the MRC/Derbyshire Smoking Study, *International Journal of Epidemiology*, *12*, 185–92.

OPCS (1987) *Smoking among secondary schoolchildren in 1986*, London: HMSO.

OPCS (1987) *Adolescent drinking*, London: HMSO.

Plant, M. A., Peck, D. F. and Samuel, E. (1985) *Alcohol, drugs and school leavers*, London: Tavistock.

Potts, H., Gillies, P. A. and Herbert, M. (1986) Adolescent smoking and opinion of cigarette advertisements, *Health Education Research Theory and Practice*, *1*, 195–201.

Tacade (1985) *Alcohol education. Syllabus 11–19*, Manchester: Tacade.

West, P. (1986) Inequalities? Social class differentials in health in youth. Paper presented to the Society for Social Medicine Conference, Leicester University, September.

Williams, R. and Gillies, P. A. (1984) Do we need objective measures to validate self-reported smoking? *Public Health*, *98*, 294–304.

11

GRAHAM HART

AIDS, HOMOSEXUAL MEN AND
BEHAVIOURAL CHANGE

Introduction

When the Acquired Immunodeficiency Syndrome (AIDS) was first recognised as a new disease entity in 1981 in the United States, homosexual men constituted 100 per cent of the identified cases. Today the majority of people infected world-wide with Human Immunodeficiency Virus (HIV), the causative agent of AIDS, are heterosexual, but in the United States and Northern Europe homosexual and bisexual men still constitute the largest groups affected by every stage of the HIV disease spectrum, from asymptomatic infection through to full-blown AIDS. These are also the risk groups amongst which the most extensive studies of behaviour and behavioural change have been taking place and it is the aim of this paper to review some of these.

Although AIDS may be a new disease, contemporary social and political reactions to it in the West are not without precedent. Alan Brandt in his study of the social history of venereal disease in the United States since 1880, *No Magic Bullet* (1987), compares late nineteenth- and early twentieth-century responses to the 'terrible peril' (Adler, 1980) wrought by syphilis and gonorrhoea to more recent cultural responses to AIDS. These include, amongst others, a pervasive fear of unrestricted contagion, panic over possible casual transmission, the stigmatization of those who are or *might* be affected (particularly appropriate when the majority of these people are constructed as sexually deviant) and, finally, heated debate and conflict over the extent to which civil liberties, particularly of the few, should be curtailed in the best interests of the wider public health. To this list one could add the process of ascribing to different groups degrees of culpability, so that prostitutes in the past and homosexual men, drug users and – once again – prostitutes today are in some way collecting their just rewards for behaviours which offend moral precepts whilst the entirely blameless (e.g. haemophiliacs or the unknowing girlfriends of bisexual men) are awarded the status of innocent victims. As Brandt makes clear, all of these responses marked attempts to deal with the major sexually transmitted diseases until at least World War II; even when treatments became available, the myths attached to, and stigma associated with, these diseases held powerful sway, particularly in the United States where there remains no federal-wide systematic public health provision for sexually transmitted diseases.

As yet there is only symptomatic treatment available to those with HIV disease and AIDS. This raises another issue on which Brandt has written. So far the only means by which an individual can protect him or herself from infection, and/or prevent the further transmission of HIV, is to pursue behaviour which avoids risk to self and others. Unfortunately, this has led to an emphasis, and sometimes exclusive focus on, individual behaviour as if that behaviour were entirely voluntaristic and free from external forces, divorced from a social context of powerful influences not all of which are subject to simple or immediate modification. We know this from research into other health-related behaviours such as smoking, alcoholism and diet, and so a model which is based purely on individual responsibility for sexual behaviour (which, it must be remembered, is also a *health* behaviour) – will have little value if no reference is made to the social, social-psychological and even economic contexts in which sexual behaviour takes place. Some of the studies reported here certainly take these and similar factors into account although unfortunately that cannot be said of them all. After reviewing the research that has been undertaken and is currently underway in relation to homosexual and bisexual men and AIDS, it is worth considering ways in which subsequent investigations of human sexual behaviour could benefit from the methodological and epistemological experience of these studies.

Studies of homosexual and bisexual behaviour

There is a strong tradition in the United States of research into homosexual and bisexual behaviour (Kinsey *et al.*, 1948; Bell and Weinberg, 1978; Gebhard and Johnson, 1979; Jay and

Young, 1979; Darrow et al., 1981). Despite the methodological criticisms levelled at these studies – mainly linked to restricted recruitment – they do provide examples of objective but sympathetic research undertaken in the pre–AIDS era; Kinsey's chapter on interviewing remains an exemplar of the execution of research in sensitive areas of human action. However, although there was often information on, for example, lifetime number of sexual partners (Bell and Weinberg, 1978; Gebhard and Johnson, 1979) detailed breakdowns of specific sexual activities – important baseline measures against which subsequent behavioural studies can be compared – were often eschewed.

It was, in fact, behavioural and epidemiological research which first indicated that AIDS might be caused by an infectious aetiological agent – subsequently to be identified as what we now know as Human Immunodeficiency Virus – and as early as 1982, Marmor et al. found an association between Kaposi's sarcoma, the major tumour of AIDS, and receptive anal intercourse. The earliest case-control studies for risk factors for AIDS had found an association with numbers of male sexual partners; more recently Moss et al. (1987) have compared AIDS cases with groups of HIV-antibody-negative neighbourhood and clinic controls in San Francisco. They found a correlation between number of sexual partners and level of risk, although receptive anal intercourse was found to be asociated with *increased* risk, *independent* of number of partners (cf. Johnson, 1987).

Although a large number of studies have now examined risk factors for HIV sero-positivity amongst homosexual and bisexual men and have reported that receptive anal intercourse is the act with the strongest independent risk for infection (Goedert et al., 1984; Melbye et al., 1984, Groopman et al., 1985; Jeffries et al., 1985; Nicholson et al., 1985; Kingsley et al., 1987; Darrow et al., 1987; Moss et al., 1987; Winkelstein et al., 1987) most of these have been purely epidemiological studies and have therefore not investigated the social context in which high-risk sexual acts have taken place. Some have not even gone so far as to describe key socio-demographic attributes of the populations studied and certainly do not make reference to such social-psychological indicators as level of knowledge, attitudes to AIDS and sexual behaviour, or subjective perceptions of risk. To be fair, this was not their aim or intention, but if we *are* properly to understand this behaviour we must look beyond the individual sexual acts: both to the objective circumstances in which they take place and to the meanings which inform these behaviours.

An early study, which began to move some way towards at least describing the participants in and the context of sexual behaviour, was undertaken in 1983 by Leon McKusick *et al.* (1985). Men were recruited in the San Francisco Bay Area from bathhouses, gay bars, through advertising in local gay newspapers for men who specifically did not frequent bars or saunas and from a group of men who were known to be in committed relationships and had participated in a previous study. In the study, 655 men completed a questionnaire on their sexual practices during the previous month in 1983 and for the same month one year before. The majority of the men in all groups were white, with a college education and incomes of between $20,000 and $30,000 per annum.

The men who regularly attended bathhouses showed little change in their frequency of bathhouse use, number of sexual partners and high–risk sexual practices such as unprotected anal intercourse over the year, whereas the other groups showed substantial reductions in terms of frequency of attendance at locations where they could meet sexual partners, number of sexual partners and the range of high-risk activities they pursued.

The study by McKusick *et al.* was one of the first to evidence a discrepancy between cognitive appreciation of risk for AIDS and actual behaviour. Although objective levels of knowledge regarding AIDS and protective health directives were reported to be high amongst all groups, subjective sexual behaviour did not change in the light of this knowledge amongst all groups. On the other hand, sexual behaviour was quite compatible with strongly held health *beliefs*. For example, 50 per cent of the bath group and 58 per cent of the bar group believed that they were in some way less susceptible to AIDS than other gay men. Again, if one focuses on the meanings which inform sexual activity, rather than on knowledge, behaviour becomes explicable in terms of these meanings. Of those men agreeing with the statement 'I use hot anonymous sex to relieve tensions', 81 per cent had had three *or more* partners during the previous month. Thus, whilst levels of knowledge may be high, other perceptions may prove more significant in explaining behaviour. Indeed, Kelly *et al.* (1987) detected no relationship at all between knowledge of risks for AIDS and behaviour. Although this was a study of homosexual men, it is unlikely that this is a finding which will be peculiar to this population, given what we know of other life-threatening behaviours such as smoking and driving at speed.

Since the paper by McKusick *et al.* was published, a number of researchers have begun to look in greater detail at social,

GRAHAM HART 131

demographic and attitudinal variables associated with behaviour and behavioural change. What are these changes, and which factors have been identified as significant in terms of explaining such changes?

All of the prospective studies which measure behaviour at one given point in time (T1) and subsequently compare this to a second point in time (T2) (Centers for Disease Control, 1985; Stevens et al., 1986; Fox et al., 1987; Van Griensven, 1987; Willoughby et al., 1987; Johnson and McGrath, 1987; Quadland et al., 1987) evidence behavioural modifications in terms of a fall in the number of sexual partners during the period of study and reductions in the level of high-risk sexual behaviour, particularly unprotected anal intercourse. This holds true regardless of the time period studied, whether this be 6 months (Siegel et al., 1987), 2 years (Joseph et al, 1987) or even 7 years, as in one cohort study (Doll et al., 1987) which collected information in 1978 before the AIDS epidemic began in San Francisco, and compared this to 1985.

Declining numbers of sexual partners range from quite small reductions – for example, from a mean of 7.7 to 6.4 partners in one Canadian study during two 6-month periods in 1984 and 1985 (Willoughby et al., 1987) – to the major change identified in the pre- and post-AIDS study in San Francisco from sixteen partners during a 4-month period in 1978 to a mean of only one in the past 4 months in 1985 (Doll et al., 1987).

In terms of high-risk sexual behaviour, studies such as that undertaken by Joseph et al. (1987), of 650 men in Chicago, show a fall from 35 per cent of men engaging in unprotected receptive anal intercourse in mid–1984 to only 6 per cent participating in this behaviour by mid–1986. Martin (1987), relying on recall of sexual activity pre- and post-AIDS, identifies a 70 per cent decline in the frequency of sexual episodes involving the exchange of body fluids and mucous-membrane contact amongst a sample of 745 men interviewed in New York in 1985.

Evidence of other positive behavioural changes include an increase in condom use by gay men (Martin, 1987; Siegel et al., 1987; Valdiserri et al., 1987) and studies which explore the roles of HIV–antibody counselling and testing in contributing to safer-sex behaviours (Coates et al., 1987; Farthing et al., 1987; Van Griensven, 1987; Willoughby et al., 1987). However, despite these generally positive trends, *all* of the studies concerned in some way with behavioural change have identified sub-groups within the study populations who either maintain, or in some cases actually begin, very high-risk activity. Are there identifiable attributes which distinguish groups pursuing safe and unsafe sexual behaviour?

Willoughby *et al.* (1987) showed that the greatest changes in behaviour were to be found amongst the 35 per cent of their total of 430 men who were antibody positive. Unfortunately, however, this meant that many of the men tested as negative continued to have high-risk sex. For example, whilst only 7 per cent of antibody-positive men reported *never* using condoms in passive anal intercourse with casual partners, 35 per cent of negatives reported such unprotected sex with casual partners. Thus, sero-negatives modified their behaviour to a lesser degree than sero-positives.

Siegel *et al.* (1987), in a longitudinal study of 161 asympto-matic men in New York, interviewed participants on two occasions 6 months apart. Men were allocated scores on the basis of their reported sexual behaviour and they were also asked for a subjec-tive rating of the riskiness of their own behaviour in terms of the likelihood of contracting and transmitting HIV. When comparing data over the 6 months, 17 per cent of the men actually increased their risk rating, and a full 41 per cent were practising risky sex at both time points. When respondents' subjective ratings of the riskiness of their behaviour were compared to their objectively allocated score, it was determined that as many as four out of five men engaging in high-risk sex may be greatly underestimating the danger inherent in that behaviour.

Unfortunately, no social, psychological or even demographic data have been presented alongside these studies to explain what, if any, features distinguish those groups who pursue or begin high-risk sexual behaviour from those who do not. Nevertheless, there clearly are identifiable groups putting themselves and oth-ers at risk of infection; other studies have demonstrated levels of risk-taking behaviour ranging from 10 per cent of a study population (Richwald *et al.*, 1987) to 40 per cent of men in one project (Quadland *et al.*, 1987) engaging in high-risk sex. A particularly worrying study (McCusker, 1987) reported that 31 per cent of a group of HIV antibody-positive men in Bos-ton reported unprotected insertive anal intercourse with multiple partners which, given the previously reported data on the role of receptive anal intercourse as the sexual behaviour associated with highest risk of viral transmission, is evidence of a failure to effect change amongst a potentially infectious group.

Happily this and other studies have attempted to investigate variables other than those that are purely behavioural. For example, Joseph *et al.* (1987) identified a group of 23 per cent of their 650 Chicago men who either consistently pursued high-risk practices, or whose behaviour in some sense 'worsened' during the period of study. They found significant differences between the high- and low-risk groups in terms of three major variables; surprisingly, given previously reported data, level of knowledge was found to be a significant factor ($p < .01-.05$) with high levels of knowledge being associated with low risk behaviour. An absence of peer norms encouraging safe sex amongst the high risk group was associated with unsafe behaviour ($p < .01-.02$) as were difficulties with sexual impulse control ($p < .01-.02$). The latter is a similar finding to the study by McKusick *et al.* (1985) in terms of the men who maintained they used 'hot anonymous sex to relieve tension'.

Another study which has explored socio-demographic as well as behavioural variables has been undertaken by Richwald *et al.* (1987) of sexual relations amongst 807 men attending seven bathhouses in Los Angeles County. Encouragingly the majority of men (61 per cent) participated only in activities associated with low risk of HIV transmission in the bathhouses, but 10 per cent engaged in such high-risk activities as active and passive anal intercourse. Comparing the two groups Richwald *et al.* found that more members of the high-risk group were significantly ($p < .05$) likely to be under 30, belong to minority groups, earn less that $20,000 per annum, have not attended college and have had five or more sexual partners during the last month. Interestingly, similar proportions reported familiarity with information in the bathhouse on AIDS (96 per cent of the high-risk group as against 98 per cent of the low-risk group) and felt it played a role in their understanding of AIDS prevention (84 per cent as against 86 per cent).

These data indicate that the majority of sexually active men who attend bathhouses in an area of the United States with a high prevalence of HIV infection amongst homosexual men are now practising low-risk sexual behaviour, but that imaginative efforts are required to direct health promotion efforts to those young, minority, low-income and less-educated men at highest risk; posters in bathhouses are a necessary but, in isolation, insufficient means of encouraging behavioural change.

Finally, and returning to the work of McKusick *et al.* (1987) data from the two large cohorts of 700 and 843 men recruited in San Francisco in 1983/4 have identified eight predictors which, at a high level of significance (p<.001), distinguish those who are not only able to pursue but to sustain low-risk activity from those who do not.

McKusick *et al.* found that *personal efficacy* – the belief that one is capable of making the recommended changes – was the variable most powerfully associated with level of risk activity. *Men in relationships*, perhaps assuming their partner to be uninfected and unlikely to sero-convert, engaged in behaviours that were most likely to transmit HIV as compared to men not in a stable relationship. Remarkably, *depression* was found to be greater amongst those who subsequently reduced their risk level. As in the Richwald *et al.* bathhouse study (1987), *younger men* were more likely to engage in high-risk activity than older men. The fifth predictor was *level of agreement with risk reduction guidelines*, with low level of agreement being associated with high-risk. Those men who *denied the virulence* of the epidemic continued to pursue high risk activity, whilst holding that a *visual image of AIDS deterioration* was related to low-risk activity. This last point matches an earlier finding of McKusick *et al.* (1985) that low-risk activity was associated with recall of seeing an AIDS patient in an advanced stage of the disease. Finally, *drug and alcohol* use during sexual activity was correlated with non-compliance with safe sex practices, a finding supported by other studies (Greenblatt, 1987; Ostrow *et al.*, 1987).

Sadly we have no data as yet from McKusick *et al.* regarding socio–demographic features of the high-risk populations, but it would be remarkable if these data did not match those presented in the Richwald *et al.* bathhouse study in terms of ethnicity, income, education and age. The McKusick *et al.* study has a heavy bias towards white, middle-class men, as do most of the studies of homosexual populations in the United States. Recruitment to these studies is often undertaken in clinics or neighbourhoods which are predominantly white and middle-class; it should also be said that many of these are longitudinal cohort studies requiring a sustained level of commitment which it may be easier to obtain from highly educated, economically secure men. These are methodological issues which it is worth considering briefly before ending.

The essential point being made here is that whilst studies which focus on behaviour alone must be seen as useful in providing some measure of, for example, the effectiveness of national and local health education initiatives, or at least of the response of specific gay communities to the arrival of HIV and AIDS, much more information needs to be collected on those factors which inform and explain behavioural change in these populations. We now know from epidemiological studies that there has been a major decline in such sexually transmitted infections as gonorrhoea amongst male homosexual clinic attenders in New York (Schultz *et al.*, 1984) and in London (Gellan and Ison, 1986; Carne *et al.*, 1987), and this is an invaluable objective indicator of changed sexual behaviour in response to the threat of HIV. But these and other purely behavioural studies will not help to direct health education efforts to those who remain at risk.

The male homosexual population in the United States turns out to be a heterogeneous group, the majority of whom *have* changed their sexual behaviour but with substantial sections continuing to pursue high-risk behaviour. This is where the studies undertaken by McKusick *et al.*, and others, can contribute to our understanding of behaviour in its social and social-psychological context. For example, findings which relate to perceived level of susceptibility to the infection and underestimations of its virulence could be exploited in appropriately tailored health-education messages, and the data on class, ethnicity and the relative youth of those most at risk incorporated into programmes – such as health outreach work – which can be targeted to groups other than those who already appear to have taken cognisance of and acted upon safe-sex messages. Research informed by a model of health behaviour which invests total responsibility for change with the individual, to the exclusion of structural and cultural constraints, is less likely to provide us with this kind of multi–layered, often complex, information which is so necessary if health promotion efforts are to achieve successful outcomes.

Conclusion

Most of the studies reported here have come from North America, with a strong representation from the east and west coasts of the continental United States. Social and behavioural research there has followed in the wake of the epidemic; political, funding and methodological issues aside, it is therefore to some extent in advance of recently begun studies in the United Kingdom. There are now two major Medical Research Council (MRC) funded studies underway in this country (Coxon, Davies and McManus; Fitzpatrick, Boulton and Hart), both of which can benefit from the experience of the American studies.

Like the American studies, the British research relies on self-reported accounts of behaviour and behavioural change, with Coxon *et al.* employing sexual diaries as the main instrument for data collection, and the Fitzpatrick *et al.* study relying on interviews in the first instance with a follow-up questionnaire one year later. Methodologically, neither approach is perfect, particularly in relation to recall of behaviour, sometimes of up to one year ago, but this is just one of a range of methodological problems faced by researchers in this field. For example, with no previous large-scale studies of sexual behaviour on which to draw when designing studies, there is no obvious sampling frame which can be used to guide recruitment to these studies. On the issue of recruitment we have as yet no idea of the extent to which it will be possible to recruit from gay pubs and clubs, through advertising in gay newspapers and magazines and through snowball recruitment, although efforts will be made in all these areas. McManus and McEvoy (1987) successfully recruited 1,292 British homosexual men to a sexual behaviour study using a self-completed postal questionnaire; however, it remains to be seen how recruitment to interviews outside the clinical context – where most of the American studies have taken place – will work out.

What one can say, however, is that these predominantly community-based studies provide opportunities to seek out and recruit men from a wide range of socio-demographic backgrounds, in relation to age, social class, ethnicity and region. Whilst the American studies have proved invaluable in terms of broad research design, they cannot be transposed unproblematically to the British scene; their restricted population in terms of social class and ethnicity alone make this impossible.

What the early and ongoing American studies and also the recently initiated British studies of homosexual behaviour can do, however, is to direct attention to key areas of investigation for the heterosexual studies which will inevitably arise as a result of predictions of the expected course of the HIV epidemic (see also Siegel and Bauman, in Feldman and Johnson (eds), 1986). In relation to non-clinic recruitment this could include targeting potential participants from known heterosexual meeting places such as 'singles' bars and night clubs, or recruiting from predominantly heterosexually active populations such as college students and members of the armed forces. Again, apart from collecting essential socio-demographic data – remarkable for their absence in some of the American studies and unwittingly reflecting heterosexual assumptions about the homogeneity of homosexual populations – one would also wish to see reference to such attitudinal variables as health beliefs regarding sexual activity and the meanings which inform sexual behaviour rather than exclusively behavioural, descriptive accounts. As McKusick and others have demonstrated, these attitudinal variables can be predictive of action and therefore invaluable when constructing health promotion strategies.

One of the aims of present and future studies of sexual behaviour – regardless of the nature of the study population – should be to produce objective data which will inform our understanding of and contribute to explanations of these behaviours. To return to points made earlier, if this aim is realised we may avoid the process of stigmatising groups at risk and thereby eschew the allocation of blame. Avoiding a blinkered focus on the indivual and his/her behaviour should also be a prerequisite of any research undertaken; otherwise the exclusion of the social and cultural forces which are the true context of sexual response will produce impoverished accounts, devoid of insight into this, apparently singular and personal, but actually overwhelmingly universal, sphere of human desire.

References

Adler, M. W. (1980) The terrible peril: a historical perspective on the venereal diseases, *Br. Med. J. 281*, 206–11.

Bell, A. P. and Weinberg, M. S. (1978) Homosexualities: a study of diversity among men and women, New York: Simon & Simon.

Brandt, A. M. (1987) *No Magic Bullet – A Social History of Venereal Disease in the United States since 1880*, Oxford: Oxford University Press.

Carne, C. A., Johnson, A. M., Pearce, F. *et al.* (1987) Prevalence of antibodies to human immunodeficiency virus, gonorrhoea rates, and changed sexual behaviour in homosexual men in London, *Lancet, i*, 656–8.

Centers for Disease Control (1985) Self-reported behavioural change among gay and bisexual men – San Francisco, *MMWR 34*, 613–15.

Coates, T. J., Morin, S. F. and McKusick, L. (1987) Consequences of AIDS antibody testing among gay men: The AIDS behavioural research project. Paper presented at the Third International Conference on AIDS, Washington.

Coxon, A. P. M., Davies, P. M. and McManus, T. J. (project in progress) A longitudinal study of the sexual behaviour of non-heterosexual males and the seroprevalence of HIV. Funding: Medical Research Council.

Darrow, W. W., Barrett, D., Jay, K. and Young A. (1981) The gay report on sexually transmitted diseases. *Am. J. Public Health 71*, 1004–11.

Darrow, W. W., Echenberg, D. F., Jaffe, H. W. *et al.* (1987) Risk Factors for human immunodeficiency virus (HIV) infection in homosexual men, *Am. J. Public Health 77*, 479–83.

Doll, L. S., Darrow, W., O'Malley, P., *et al* (1987) Self-reported behavioural change in homosexual men in the San Francisco city clinic cohort. Paper presented at the Third International Conference on AIDS, Washington.

Farthing, C. F., Jesson, W., Taylor, H. L. *et al.* (1987) The HIV antibody test: influence on sexual behaviour of homosexual men, Paper presented at the Third International Conference on AIDS, Washington.

Feldman, D. A. and Johnson, T. (eds) (1986) *The Social dimensions of AIDS: Method and theory*, New York: Praeger.

Fitzpatrick, R., Boulton, M. and Hart, G. (project in progress) The health beliefs and health behaviour of male homosexuals in relation to AIDS. Funding: Medical Research Council.

Fox, R., Ostrow, D., Valdiserri, M. *et al.* (1987) Changes in sexual activities in the multicentre AIDS cohort study, Paper presented at the Third International Conference on AIDS, Washington.

Gebhard, P. H. and Johnson, A. B. (1979) *The Kinsey Data: Marginal Tabulations of the 1938–1963 Interviews Conducted by the Institute for Sex Research*, Philadelphia: W. B. Saunders.

Gellan, M. C. A. and Ison, C. A. (1986) Declining incidence of gonorrhoea in London: a response to fear of AIDS? *Lancet ii*, 920.

Goedert, J. J., Biggar, R. J., Winn, D. M. *et al.* (1984) Determinants of retrovirus (HTLV III) antibody and immunideficiency conditions in homosexual men, *Lancet, ii*, 711–16.

Greenblatt, R. M., Samuel, M., Osmond, D. *et al.* (1987) Risk factors for seroconversion with human immunodeficiency virus among homosexual men in San Francisco. Paper presented at the Third International Conference on AIDS, Washington.

Groopman, J. E., Mayer, K. H., Sarngadharan, M. G. *et al.* (1985) Seroepidemiology of human T-Lymphotropic virus type III among homosexuals with the acquired immunodeficiency syndrome or generalised lymphadenopathy and among asymptomatic controls in Boston. Ann. Intern. Med. *102*, 334–7.

Jay, K. and Young, A. (1979) *The Gay Report*, New York: Summit.

Jeffries, E., Willoughby, K. B., Boyko, W. *et al.* (1985) The Vancouver lymphadenopathy AIDS study: seroepidemiology of HTLV III antibody, *Can. Med. Assoc. J. 132*, 1373–7.

Johnson, A. M. (1988) Social and behavioural aspects of the HIV epidemic – a review, *J. Roy Statist. Soc.* (in press).

Johnson, D. and McGrath, H. M. (1987) Perceived changes in sexual practices among homosexual men, Paper presented at the Third International Conference on AIDS, Washington.

Joseph, J.G., Montgomery, S., Kessler, R. C. *et al.* (1987) Two-year
   longitudinal study of behavioural risk reduction in a cohort of homosexual men, Paper presented at the Third International Conference
   on AIDS, Washington.
Kelly, J. A., St Lawrence, J. S., Brasfield, T. L. and Hood, H. V.
   (1987) Relationships between knowledge about AIDS and actual
   behaviour in a sample of homosexual men: some implications for
   prevention, Paper presented at the Third International Conference
   on AIDS, Washington.
Kingsley, L. A., Detels, R., Kaslow, R. *et al.* (1987) Risk factors
   for seroconversion to human immunodeficiency virus among male
   homosexuals, *Lancet, i*, 345–8.
Kinsey, A. C., Pomeroy, W. B. and Martin, C. E. (1948) Sexual
   behaviour in the human male, Philadelphia: W.B. Sanders.
McCusker, J., Zapka, J. G., Stoddard, A. M. *et al.* (1987) Determinants
   and effects of HIV antibody test disclosure, Paper presented at the
   Third International Conference on AIDS, Washington.
McKusick, L., Coates, T. J., Wiley, J. A. *et al.* (1987) Prevention
   of HIV infection among gay and bisexual men: two longitudinal
   studies, Paper presented at the Third International Conference on
   AIDS, Washington.
McKusick, L., Horstman, W. and Coates, T. J. (1985) AIDS and sexual
   behaviour reported by gay men in San Francisco, *Am. J. Public Health*
   75, 4933–96.
McManus, T. J. and McEvoy, M. (1987) Some aspects of male homosexual behaviour in the United Kingdom, *Br. J. Sexual Medicine*,
   110–20.
Marmor, M., Friedman-Kien, A. E., Laubenstein, L. *et al.* (1982)
   Risk factors for Kaposi's sarcoma in homosexual men, *Lancet, i*,
   1083–7.
Martin, J. L. (1987) The impact of AIDS on gay male sexual behaviour
   patterns in New York City, *Am. J. Public Health, 77*, 578–81.
Melbye, M., Biggar, R. J., Ebbesen, P. *et al.* (1984) Seroepidemiology
   of HTLV III in Danish homosexual men; prevalence, transmission
   and disease outcome, *Br. Med. J. 289*, 573–5.
Moss, A. R., Osmond, D., Bacchetti, P. *et al.* (1987) Risk factors for
   AIDS and HIV seropositivity in homosexual men, *Am. J. Epidemiology, 125*, 1035–47.
Nicholson, J. K., McDougal, J. S., Jaffe, H. W. *et al.* (1985) Exposure
   to human T-lymphoropic virus type III/Lymphadenopathy-associated
   virus and immunologic abnormalities in asymptomatic homosexual
   men, *Ann. Intern. Med. 103*, 37–42.
Ostrow, D. G., Van Raden, M., Kingsley, L. *et al.* (1987) Drug
   use and sexual behaviour change in a cohort of homosexual men,
   Paper presented at the Third International Conference on AIDS,
   Washington.
Quadland, M., Shattls, W. D., Schuman, R. and Jacobs, R. (1987)

The 800 men study: a controlled study of an AIDS prevention program in New York City. Paper presented at the Third International Conference on AIDS, Washington.

Richwald, G. A., Kristal, A. R., Kyle, G. R. *et al.* (1987) Sexual relations in bathhouses in Los Angeles County: implications for AIDS prevention education, Paper presented at the Third International Conference on AIDS, Washington.

Schultz, S., Friedman, S., Kristal, A. *et al.* (1984) Declining rates of rectal and pharyngeal gonorrhoea among men – New York City. *JAMA, 252,* 327.

Siegel, K., Chen, J. Y., Meragno, F. and Christ, G. (1987) Persistence and change in sexual behaviour and perceptions of risk for AIDS among homosexual men, Paper presented at the Third International Conference on AIDS, Washington.

Stevens, C. E., Taylor, P. E., Zang, E. A. *et al.* (1986) Human T-Cell lymphotropic virus type III infection in a cohort of homosexual men in New York City, *JAMA, 225,* 2167–72.

Valdiserri, R. O., Lyter, D., Callahan, C. *et al.* (1987) Condom use in a cohort of gay and bisexual men, Paper presented at the Third International Conference on AIDS, Washington.

Van Griensven, G. J. P., Tielman, R. A. P., Goudsmit, J. *et al.* (1987) Effect of HIV ab serodiagnosis on sexual behaviour in homosexual men in the Netherlands, Paper presented at the Third International Conference on AIDS, Washington.

Willoughby, R., Schecter, M. T., Boyko, W. J. *et al.* (1987) Sexual practices and condom use in a cohort of homosexual men: evidence of differential modification between seropositive and seronegative men, Paper presented at the Third International Conference on AIDS, Washington.

Winkelstein, W., Lyman, D. M., Padian, N. *et al.* (1987) Sexual practices and risk of infection by the human immunodeficiency virus, *JAMA, 257,* 312–25.

12

KATHRYN BACKETT

PUBLIC HEALTH AND PRIVATE LIVES

Introduction

In recent years there has been increasing acknowledgement of the need for public health research which will enable greater understanding of the social processes and factors involved in the development of health-related behaviours. For example, little is known about the everyday social contexts which are conducive or detrimental to health; and particularly how lay people themselves perceive health and illness and their place generally in life.

The dearth of this kind of information may be attributed partly to the dominance of biomedically based large-scale surveys in public health research. Such methods provide aggregate data which demonstrate statistical associations between demographic variables and aspects of physical and mental health and illness. However, they do not explain how such variables interact dynamically at the individual or family level and, therefore, how health may be understood as one component of ordinary daily life (MacIntyre, 1986).

In this chapter it is argued that public health research should examine those aspects of daily life which enable people to be healthy as well as those which make them sick. Furthermore, health-related behaviours should be studied not simply as individually determined but rather as social products which are subject to complex structural and interactional constraints.

141

*Everyday health in families – some methodological
and theoretical concerns in a current study*

A study currently in progress at the Research Unit in Health and
Behavioural Change is addressing some of these shortfalls in public
health research. It is a multi-interview qualitative study which is
exploring the everyday lives and health-related behaviours of a
sample of married couples with two children aged between 3 and 10
years. Spouses are being interviewed individually and jointly four
times over an 18-month field-work period.

A sample was drawn from the records of an Edinburgh group
general practice serving a predominantly middle-class area of the
city. Initially every couple was selected who met the following
criteria: they were private home-owners; they had one or both
partners in non-manual occupations; they did not have a family
member suffering *chronic* physical, mental or social problems;
and, by virtue of having children in the designated age group, they
were at a similar point in the life course. Following a random selection procedure twenty-eight families were recruited. This small
homogeneous sample is characterised by being in broadly similar
material and social circumstances. These are such that, theoretically, respondents are well-placed in socio-economic terms to lead
'healthy' lives. Moreover, in statistical terms, these respondents
fit into groups with a lower probability of contracting many of
the major chronic diseases common to western societies. Detailed
qualitative interviews are examining in depth the similarities and
differences in health beliefs and behaviours of this sample. In particular, the interviews are focusing on respondents' accounts of the
processes, contexts and 'strategies' (Lofland, 1976) involved in
everyday health-related behaviours.

A major aim of this study is to move away from the restrictions
of the biomedically-based pathogenic approach to investigating
health and illness. Taking a 'salutogenic' approach and 'studying
health instead of disease' (Antonovsky, 1979), involves asking
different kinds of questions and experimenting with different
methodologies. The salutogenic approach assumes that health and
illness are not dichotomous entities but points on a multi-
dimensional continuum. Moreover, emphasis is placed on the
importance of studying subjective interpretations of health and
illness; and these may or may not be directly related to biomedically defined physiological states.

Thus, the adoption of a salutogenic approach necessitates the
broadening of parameters of interest in order to understand, *within*

their relevant social contexts, behaviours which may have implications for health. In the present study it was decided to locate individuals principally in their domestic lives since this is the arena for much primary health and illness care. Influenced by interactionist and phenomenological theory (Blumer, 1969; Schutz, 1972) the research aims to uncover how respondents themselves view health, and its place in their lives. The exploratory nature of the study, employing semi-structured qualitative interviewing techniques, means that the researcher encourages respondents themselves to identify and discuss items which may have implications for their health on an everyday basis. Meeting respondents several times in their own homes and stressing the importance of respondents' own ideas about health facilitates the development of what Lofland (1976) has called 'intimate familiarity'.

Analysis of data is an integral part of the field-work in this study. Themes arising from interviews are systematically identified and then assembled (Lofland, 1976). Techniques of 'grounded theory development' (Glaser and Strauss, 1968) are also being used. Here theory and method are interconnected since the multi-interview study enables the researcher to tease out concepts, check these against data, further explore data which seem to be exceptional cases, and also go back to respondents in order to refine concepts and theories (Filstead, 1970; Schatzman, 1973; Lofland, 1971). In this way the research process becomes focused on the *generation* rather than the *testing* of theory. Glaser and Strauss (1967) said that, in this way:

. . . grounded theories can emerge which instead of forcing data into preconceived 'objective' reality, seek to mobilise as a research tool the categories which the participants themselves use to order their experience.

The value of grounded theory research for health education research (and by extension public health research generally) has been propounded by Mullen and Reynolds (1978). Amongst other points they stressed that researchers have often, 'not made a significant commitment to leaving open a redefinition of the problem'. Thus, in the present study, concepts and ideas as they emerge from respondents' accounts are systematically recorded, classified and cross-referenced. The analysis involves an immersion in the data, ideally achieved, as in this study, by the researcher being both interviewer and analyst.

However, making the transition from studying public health at the population level to exploring everyday health-related behaviours in the private arena of domestic life is very much more complex than merely adopting an alternative theoretical perspective and experimenting with different methodologies. Many of the complexities apply to any sociological endeavour, but some are particularly pertinent to studying domestically-based relationships, in this case families. In such relationships there are cross-cutting demands of institutional, normative and personal expectations. Also, in addition to the power struggles characterising any social group, the development of familial behaviours is complicated by the expectation of emotional commitment. Research difficulties are further compounded by such behaviours being called 'private life', and thus accorded a degree of socially-sanctioned impenetrability! For the researcher this creates special problems of access which may not be experienced so acutely in other studies of human groups . Such problems are evidenced methodologically. For instance, direct observation is difficult and full of methodological problems; participant observation is, by definition, impossible; enlisting key informants to report on the group's behaviours is probably biased and may be damaging or even unethical; self-reporting is especially insightful only if all group members co-operate and do so independently of one another. Ideally interviews should take place with all family members. This, added to the usual problems of reliability and validity, may result in particular difficulties in recruiting respondents.

Issues of domestic privacy are further complicated by the very taken-for-grantedness of people's daily lives. Moreover, several researchers have suggested that respondents find it difficult to talk about their 'health'; and that 'illness', being a more problematical state, has proved easier to address for *all* concerned (Locker, 1981; Blaxter and Paterson, 1982). Cornwell (1984) found that her working class respondents talked about health and illness in two main ways. Firstly they put forward what she called 'public accounts' which focused largely on moral and evaluative aspects of health and illness, and drew heavily on what were believed to be *medically* acceptable theories and concepts. Often these accounts were expressed as something separate or abstracted from personal experience. Secondly, however, respondents put forward 'private accounts' which included much more practical and pragmatic experiences and were *less* concerned with social or moral 'public' acceptability. These accounts were often expressed in the form of story-telling or relating personal experiences. This is a useful distinction for those involved with public health if only because it raises the question: which of these accounts is the more meaningful for actual behaviours? Perhaps it might be suggested that public accounts reflect broadly based 'oughts' of behaviour, whereas private accounts explain individual interpretations of these 'oughts' and how they are, or are not, realised in everyday behaviours.

The distinction also has considerable implications for public health research. It seems that public accounts are more likely to be given in one-off standardised interviews, particularly those where few open-ended questions are included. Such methods still provide the backbone of much public health research. If it is thought that these kinds of responses accurately reflect and predict health-related behaviours then no further developments are necessary. But predicting health-related behaviours on the basis of such data has proved notoriously difficult, as has changing behaviours through health-education (Gatherer, 1979; Wenzel, 1983; Hunt and Martin, 1988). Other social and psychological forces seem to be at work which may or may not influence behaviours in ways seen as acceptable by those interested in a particular public health issue. If, as seems intuitively plausible, private accounts *are* more directly reflective of actual behaviours then appropriate research methodologies to provide data for those working in public health must be developed.

Study interests of particular relevance to public health

The choice of a middle-class sample. On a population level, compared with lower socio-economic groups, the middle class have lower overall mortality and morbidity rates, lower use of formal health services, and higher uptake of preventive services, although they tend to have higher general practitioner consultation rates for their children (Townsend and Davidson, 1982; Whitehead, 1987; Blaxter, 1981). It is important to note, however, that aggregating data from social classes may obscure some important variations within 'the middle class' (Brotherstone, 1976; Rose and Marmot, 1981). It could be argued therefore that whilst these groups may tend to give similar replies to questions about health, the relationship of these replies to actual health behaviours and health status is much more problematical. Nevertheless, in the present study it is hypothesised that such a group will be likely to have a positive view of health; to be receptive to health education messages; to be less likely to engage in biomedically defined health-damaging behaviours; and to have sufficient material resources to provide an environment conducive to health promoting practices.

In order to explore these hypotheses, qualitative work is necessary to clarify the social processes, contexts and meanings which underlie the statistical associations (WHO Vienna Dialogue, 1986). This is particularly pressing for those concerned about public health since much health policy is based on assumptions not only about what goes on in families but also on what 'the family' actually is. Graham (1984) has pointed out that, in particular, health policies 'presume an understanding of how families work to promote and protect the health of their members' (p. 18). However, although western society is now characterised by diversity in family forms, decisions may still be being made using, albeit implicitly, the model of the traditional nuclear family of male breadwinner and dependent wife with two children. The sample of families in the present study is therefore particularly interesting as in some respects it *does* reflect this traditional family stereotype, although two-thirds of the women are also in paid employment. An important study interest, therefore, is whether or not the presumed beliefs and behaviours related to health do in fact characterise even the kind of families which, arguably, provide an implicit model behind health policy and health education.

Studying family groups. Health beliefs and behaviours do not develop in a social vacuum. They are the outcome of structural conditions and everyday interactions. Research into family groups provides a particularly rich source of health data for a variety of reasons. For instance, study of these everyday caring behaviours within the family context allows empirical information to be gathered about health decisions and their relevance to self-care (Levin, Katz and Holst, 1977) and factors affecting the process of seeking professional medical help (Zola, 1973; Stimson and Webb, 1975). More broadly, studying domestic life provides useful data about everyday interactions and decision-making as these relate to health. It may be argued that family groups have a special degree of access to health knowledge about their members. Not only do they possess biographical knowledge about one another's health and illness; but there is also a high degree of visibility of behaviours within the home.

However, it is also important to query the presumed homogeneity of the health experiences of members of the same family group (Backett, 1989). Whilst it is accepted that families in different social classes may experience inequalities in health (Marmot and McDowell, 1986; Townsend and Davidson, 1982), less attention has been paid to differing patterns of health experiences and attitudes *within* a family. In part little intra-familial data exist because of the tendency to formulate different research questions about men's and women's health. Moreover, data about families have often been gathered only from one member (usually the woman), thus giving a perhaps false impression of familial consensus on health. Most often men's health issues have been related to differences in *mortality* and the public material world of the labour market, whilst study of women's health issues has concentrated on *morbidity* and sought explanation in the private social world of the family (Verbrugge, 1985; Popay, 1986; Blaxter, 1986). This must also reflect the legacy of structural functionalist approaches to the family. In the present study men and women are located in their domestic and family contexts, but account is also taken of occupational influences of *both* spouses. Feminist critiques have also drawn attention to the differential distribution of resources within families (Pahl, 1983; Brannen and Wilson, 1987); and the ways in which power relations between husbands and wives might affect health-related behaviours, for example, feeding the family (Charles and Kerr, 1987). Thus it is important for an informed public health to examine whether or not individuals in a family share the same standard of living or even lifestyle (Bernard, 1973; Backett, 1989) and if, as has been suggested, women may be particularly disadvantaged (Graham, 1984).

Gender and health. A further implication of these critiques is that research is also needed to help understand the social processes which lie behind the well established statistical associations between gender and health. Verbrugge (1985) expressed morbidity differences in terms of an iceberg with the tip representing the more potentially fatal conditions most characteristic of males, and the broad base representing the bulk of less life-threatening conditions and being predominantly female. However more information is required about the ways in which men's and women's daily lives might contribute to this vivid picture (Gove and Hughes, 1979; Arber *et al.*, 1985).

Lay health beliefs. Much health education and health promotion proceeds on the assumption that, given information, people will be 'enabled' to achieve 'healthier lifestyles'. Moreover, implicit health policy in Great Britain also assumes that the public *will* accept responsibility for their own health, particularly in the form of adopting individual preventive health practices. Such assumptions, which tend to detach 'health' from 'life circumstances', have yet to be proven empirically.

Issues such as these have begun to be addressed by researchers interested in lay health beliefs (Calnan and Johnson, 1985; Pill and Stott, 1985; Hunt and McLeod, 1987). They are demonstrating that, as anthropologists have shown in different cultures, alternative and powerful systems of health beliefs can exist alongside the dominant ideology (for detailed discussion see RUHBC, 1988, Chapter 3). In the present study the dominant ideology is western biomedicine.

The importance of social context in understanding health-related behaviours: some illustrations from the current study

Themes are already emerging during the present study which have implications for public health research. Some of these will be discussed which illustrate the importance of understanding the social contexts in which behaviours with implications for health are developed. Data are drawn from the first-round individual interviews and many of these themes are being further investigated empirically.

First, how do these respondents react to ideas about healthy living generally, and health education messages in particular? It was interesting to note that respondents often spontaneously related their own perceived good health and potential for healthy living to their relatively fortunate circumstances. Almost everyone said they considered themselves 'lucky' to live in a comfortable house in a pleasant area, and to have enough money to afford good food and a comfortable way of life. They contrasted themselves with people living in poverty, and the stresses and strains that this must impose on health. Respondents by and large found it unsurprising that people surviving unemployment and living on the breadline might not be particularly receptive to health education messages. As one man explained:

> If people are happy and content relatively with what they've got, and they've got a job and they've got a reasonable standard of living, then they're going to be more receptive to the preventive measures that are being attempted at the moment. But if you're unemployed and sitting in the middle of Pilton (deprived area of city) you're not going to be really worried about, em, a balanced diet and all the rest of it, not smoking and so on.

Not only did respondents account for good health in terms of *present* social circumstances but they also saw *ideas* about health as dynamic. They saw such ideas as a product of their time and as reflecting the socially approved 'knowledge' currently available. This was best illustrated when they were asked to reflect on their parents' views on health when they were children. The majority of respondents in fact felt that these were somewhat different from their own views. However, any criticisms of their parents were usually couched in an appreciation of the different social attitudes and possibilities prevailing at that time. As one woman said:

> It was great to be out of rationing and my father paid the meat bills, and we ate an awful lot of meat when I think back on it. And generally we ate a lot, when you were saying have I changed my habits?, I mean when I was a child I was fat and I'm still quite sturdy, but er, in proportion I'm thinner now than I was then. Er, yes we ate a lot and my children don't eat as much (they don't?) no. For breakfast they'll have a cereal and toast but we always had something hot and we would have a cooked lunch and a cooked tea and probably afternoon tea, we'd have kind of afternoon tea when we came in from school. And there was always masses of food on the go and a lot of it was a lot of milk and butter and meat (yes) which my mother thought was good for us (yes, I see) and which I don't blame her for at all. I think probably in that situation, at that time, I would have done just the same.

Others explained, however, that *their* own parents had been in much poorer circumstances than they are themselves and, again, related their parents' behaviour to this social context. Another woman said of her parents' views on health:

> They didn't have any views, I would say. I think the trouble was they didn't have any money. So, er, makes a difference, it does. They had to feed you with, that's why all this fat, this stodge – to fill you up. My dad was a miner, and, er, they weren't well paid then. And it was just a case of – you got mounds of potatoes, mounds of bread, er, all the things that were filling and cheap, you know. Sausages, that sort of thing.

A man gave the following very typical assessment of the different health-related behaviours of his parents, he said:

> I think it's just days gone by they were naïve. At that time I think they thought they were doing you good because that's what the doctors and everyone said was good for you (yes).

Thus respondents perceived generational changes in the social acceptability of behaviours related to health. They also identified many social changes in behaviours such as smoking, taking exercise and the kinds of foods eaten. However, they were in fact much more ambivalent in their *assessment* of these perceived changes; and also in how they felt about current health education messages. Often, for example, respondents might describe in some detail how their parents' past and present lifestyles were 'unhealthy' by modern standards. Then, however, they might also describe their parents' continuing good health despite *all*, and occasionally confess to some confusion about what to conclude. As one woman said:

> My mum has the most unhealthy diet (does she?) you can ever imagine. Em, and yet you know *she's still going strong in her late 60's*, smokes and eats lots of fat, you know (laughs).

Her husband, who was very much more critical of his own parents' behaviours, still acknowledged that *they* themselves felt that *their* past behaviours were not harmful. He said:

> I behave totally different. I mean my parents' view of health is 'well, if *they* had their way you wouldn't be eating anything'. Or, er, you see, the new views on diet and health and so on has directly challenged their diet, challenged it right down to the bottom, you know. Em, I mean my parents overcook vegetables, they eat too much fat, em, the diet isn't balanced, well, they're both ex-smokers, but they don't smoke anymore. Em, probably they eat too much sugar and so on, em. *And they are perfectly healthy on it*, so they don't see any reason why. It's like the old chestnut, there was an old man who smoked thirty a day until he was ninety-five and got run over by a bus. But, er, no, I behave totally different, and when they come up here it's a bit difficult.

Another woman, also from a mining background, again saw health as reflecting social circumstances perhaps as much as it did individual behaviours, she said of her parents' 'unhealthy' lifestyle:

> *I don't know if it's made that much difference at the end of the day*. But I think it's just a way of life. . . . My father's health is maybe a bit poor, but I think maybe that is the result of being a miner as much as the fact that, you know, he doesn't do any keep-fit or, you know, maybe smoking hasn't helped either. I think it's just a different way of life, a different outlook in life that we've got. I think we've got more money to sort of spend on doing activities like that and maybe they hadn't any.

Reactions to health education messages appeared also to be somewhat contradictory. Most respondents expressed some interest in watching television programmes about health, or reading such articles in newspapers or magazines. However, a sizeable minority said such things did not interest them very much at all. Most of these 'uninterested' were men, and the following comment was typical. One man said he read articles about health, 'very occasionally. Not as a priority. Given the choice of, you know, sport, financial page, general news, it might come after that.'

Others commented that they only bothered to read articles which had some particular relevance to themselves or their family. Even those who said they *did* take an active interest in health information, nevertheless expressed considerable ambivalence about its effects on their ideas or on behaviours. A man who was perhaps one of those in the sample most conscious of adopting preventive health measures claimed:

> I try to, I take on board most things that people tell you, whether or not I actually do anything about it, most things that research tells us, em. So, yes, I mean my ideas on health have changed with increasing scientific knowledge.

Nevertheless, this man, like everyone else in the sample saw a great difference between ideas and their translation into *practice* and commented, for example:

> In order to lose a stone I'd have to em, have to stop doing things that I enjoy doing, so I'm quite happy as I am.

Such comments were typical, as were these from another man who explained:

> You can find out perhaps that there are lots of things that I could be doing that could be healthier. But at the same time I have lived so far and I feel healthy and generally feel good. And, em, I'm probably doing all kinds of things wrong, but it would take an awful lot to get me motivated beyond the point that I am already.

The majority of women, although they might acknowledge actually spending more time accumulating knowledge about good health, and discussing this with friends, still emphasised the difficulties in translating this information into behaviour. Again, the following views expressed by one of the women, reflected these of many of the sample; she said:

> Well I think if I feel it can fit into my lifestyle, my way of living, then I would probably take it on. But, you know, there is sort of other things that, you know, like eating fish three times a week, and white meat three times a week, and red meat only once a week, you know. I think 'no way', you know, the children don't like fish that much and even chicken.

She went on to say that she might occasionally try dietary changes but that they all 'probably end up just kind of eating the things that you have become used to, and, you know, the children will eat.'

Analysis of the first round of field-work data suggests that even amongst groups who are aware of health education messages, considerable ambivalence exists about putting ideas into practice. Taken to its extreme, at times it appeared to the researcher that the mere *possession* of health knowledge was, *in itself*, felt by some respondents to indicate good health, whether or not this knowledge was translated into 'healthy' behaviours! As might be expected, this middle-class group of the population *has* absorbed much information about preventive health measures. Particularly in the first interviews, respondents were skilled at presenting the 'public account' of what they were *aware* should be done for good health. However, as further detail is being gathered about what actually happens in their everyday lives, a somewhat different picture is emerging.

There is also a definite scepticism about, as respondents would say, 'going overboard' and embracing new health practices. This is in part because many of these respondents perceived health education messages as often changing when new research is reported. Their ambivalence may be seen as reflecting contradictory knowledge. For example, one woman described how she often found dietary information to be somewhat confusing. She said:

> I think it is very difficult nowadays because you've been brought up to eat a certain type of food all your life, and then all of a sudden you've got a family, and somebody's telling you you have to eat this and they have to have that. And then somebody else is saying 'don't give them too many dairy foods', and if they don't get enough calcium, the only place you get it is dairy foods, you know, it can be really I think difficult.

In addition, even amongst this middle-class group, there are problems in making an act of faith that adopting a certain preventive measure will result in an eventual long term pay-off. For these reasons, and many others, most respondents were continuing to 'enjoy' things at present which they knew might be 'bad' for them in the future.

Thus the present study re-emphasises the importance for those interested in the public health critically to distinguish between receptiveness to health education messages and their translation into behavioural practice. The study is also investigating how factors in people's daily lives, perhaps not directly associated with health, affect behaviours which may have health implications. The research suggests that, in part, such factors are connected with respondents' perceptions of health, and the place of health concerns in their lives. Also, however, social and interactional constraints exist in respondents' lives which in themselves affect health-related behaviours.

It was evident from the interviews that a 'healthy life' was, in the abstract, viewed as a generally desirable state. However, the everyday ingredients of a 'healthy life' were much more difficult to describe, and were subject to quite complex positive and negative evaluations. For example, most respondents described 'a healthy life' as involving social, mental and spiritual components; and these may in themselves be seen to conflict with purely biomedically defined health. Thus, the well-worn contradiction that something 'bad' for you may do you 'good' by making you 'feel better'.

The majority of respondents found it difficult or impossible to describe someone known to them whom they saw as leading 'a healthy life'. They found it much easier to describe someone leading 'an unhealthy life' but frequently guilt was expressed about such statements which were construed as criticisms. Moral evaluation is thus an integral part of talking about health. As one man reflected when asked these questions: 'Someone who leads a healthy life, always does the right things? Right pain in the neck!.'

Moreover, if respondents *did* describe someone who led 'a healthy life' they often concluded that, whilst the person *appeared* to be doing all the 'right things' for their physical health, he or she might be in some way suspect in their social or emotional life. The active pursuit of good health could be open to moral criticism if, for example, it detracted from perceived social or familial obligations. The following quotation illustrates the kinds of reservations regularly expressed about someone who was viewed as leading 'a healthy life'. One woman said:

> That's very hard because I know a lot of people who are physically very healthy but I would not swop places with them, em, because I don't think they've got the rest of their lives sorted out. They're sort of manic about physical fitness and diet and things.'

Respondents' accounts therefore indicated that whilst a concern with physiological health might be of importance, 'good health' was seen as, in practice, a very much broader and more complex issue. A man considered the issues as follows:

> I can't think of anybody leading a healthy life (can you not?). I think I'm probably looking for someone who is the epitome of taking a lot of exercise, em, eating the right kinds of food, probably working the right hours, em, getting the mix between work and family life right, all these sort of things. I'm not sure I can think of anybody.

Therefore, for these respondents, health concerns were simply one of many competing priorities in their everyday lives. Moreover, at their current stage in the life-course, good health was taken for granted by most of them and, as such, was seldom experienced as a pressing concern. Hunt's (1987) comments aptly reflects the overall impression given by this sample. She said: 'The healthy body/mind does not demand conscious attention and the focus is outward not inward' (p. 6). In addition, the few respondents who *had* experienced some acute physical or emotional health problems appeared to have relegated these also to the taken-for-granted sphere. They indicated that they largely ignored the problems and gave the impression that these were not to the forefront of daily considerations. One man regarded his damaged back as simply something he lived with and said there was no time in his life to carry out any therapeutic exercise. Another, who had arthritic knees as a consquence of athletic injuries in his youth, also made light of these and did not do the medically prescribed exercises.

Those concerned with health promotion should acknowledge, therefore, that the individual's evaluation of the importance of health considerations takes place in the context of other demands and rewards in his/her life generally. Equally, behaviours with implications for health were often carried out, or not, for reasons which in respondents' accounts bore little direct relationship to a concern for biomedically-defined health.

To cite a few examples from the interviews: 'snack' or convenience meals were presented as an integral part of a lifestyle comprising demanding adult work schedules and busy children's play schedules; continuous car use was viewed by the majority of women as an undesirable necessity which enabled them to fit in their working lives with childcare commitments; organised exercise in leisure time was seen as facilitating relaxation and stress relief as well as promoting fitness, and was therefore appropriately followed by social drinking.

In addition, respondents regularly cited social and interactional pressures as factors which frustrated attempts to achieve 'a healthy lifestyle'. The demands on time and energy of work and familial responsibilities were the most commonly cited pressures. The ways in which such pressures impact differently on women's and men's lives are discussed in detail elsewhere (Backett, 1989). In a general sense, however, 'healthy' choices were presented by respondents as requiring an *individual* commitment or effort which was felt to be impossible because of other *social* constraints. Some illustrations occurred regularly in respondents' accounts. One example was that of the women who had regularly taken exercise before they had children, almost all found this to be extremely difficult once they had pre-nursery children. Another example concerned decisions about what to eat. These decisions were regularly affected by factors such as children's fads, whether or not *all* family members were present at the meal, and if the food had to be either rapidly prepared and/or consumed in between other social commitments.

In order better to understand health-related behaviours it is crucial then to analyse them as complex social products. It is unrealistic to view such behaviours as the responsibility of an individual living, as it were, in a social vacuum. Moreover, the present study is indicating that, even amongst groups with relatively high level of socio-economic security and health awareness, so called 'healthy' choices are by no means automatically assured.

Acknowledgements

The author wishes to acknowledge the financial support of the Scottish Health Education Group in the preparation of this work.

References

Antonovsky, A. (1979) *Health, Stress and Coping*, San Francisco, Washington and London: Jossey-Bass Publishers.
Arber, S., Gilbert, N. G. and Dale, A. (1985) Paid employment and women's health: a benefit or a source of strain?, *Sociol. Hlth and Illness* 7 (3), 375–400.
Backett, K.C. (1989) *Studying Health in Families* (Provisional title), in Cunningham-Burley, S. and McKeganey, N. P. (eds), *Readings in Medical Sociology*, London, New York: Tavistock Publications.
Bernard, J. (1973) *The Future of Marriage*, London: Souvenir Press.
Blaxter, M. (1981) *The Health of the Children*, London: Heinemann Educational Books.
Blaxter, M. (1986) A Comparison of Measures of Inequality in Morbidity, Paper presented to *ESF/ESRC Workshop on Inequalities in Health*, London: The City University.
Blaxter, M. and Paterson, E. (1982) *Mothers and Daughters: A Three Generational Study of Health Attitudes and Behaviour*, London: Heinemann Educational Books.
Blumer, H. S. (1969) *Symbolic Interactionism: Perspective and Method*, Englewood Cliffs, N.J.: Prentice-Hall Inc.
Brannen, J. and Wilson, G. (1987) *Give and Take in Families: Studies in Resource Distribution*, London: Allen & Unwin.
Brotherstone, Sir J. (1976) Inequality: Is it inevitable? The Galton

Lecture 1975, in Carter, C. O. and Peel, J. (eds) *Equalities and Inequalities in Health*, London: Academic Press, 73–104.

Calnan, M. and Johnson, B. (1985) Health, Health Risks and Inequalities: an exploratory study of women's perceptions, *Sociol. Hlth and Illness* 7 (1), 55–75.

Charles, N. and Kerr, M. (1987) Just the way it is: gender and age differences in family food consumption, in Brannen, J. and Wilson, G. (eds) *Give and Take in Families*, London: Allen & Unwin.

Cornwell, J. (1984) *Hard Earned Lives: Accounts of Health and Illness from East London*, London, New York: Tavistock Publications.

Filstead, W. J. (ed.) (1970) *Qualitative Methodology: Firsthand Involvement with the Social World*, Chicago, New York: Markham Publishing Co.

Gatherer, A., Parfit, J., Porter, E. and Vessey, E. Y. M. (1979) *Is Health Education Effective? An overview of evaluative studies*, London: Health Education Council.

Glaser, B. G. and Strauss, A. L. (1967) *The Discovery of Grounded Theory*, Chicago: Aldine Publishing Co.

Graham, H. (1984) *Women, Health and the Family*, Brighton, Eng.: Wheatsheaf Books Ltd, Harvester Press Group.

Gove, W. R. and Hughes, M. (1979) Possible causes for the apparent sex differences in physical health: an empirical investigation, *Am. J. Sociol. 44*, 126–46.

Hunt, S. M. (1987) Subjective Indicators for Health Promotion Research, Research Unit in Health and Behavioural Change, Working Paper 18, Edinburgh: Research Unit in Health and Behavioural Change.

Hunt, S. M. and McLeod, M. (1987) Health and Behavioural Change: some lay perspectives, *Comm. Med.* 9, 68–76.

Hunt, S. M. and Martin, C. J. (1988) Health related behavioural change: a test of a new model, *Psychology and Health*, *2*, 209–30.

Levin, L. S., Katz, A. M. and Holst, E. (1977) *Self Care: Lay Initiatives in Health*, London: Croom Helm.

Locker, D. (1981) *Symptoms and Illness: The Cognitive Organisation of Disorder*, London, New York: Tavistock Publications.

Lofland, J. (1971) *Analysing Social Settings: A Guide to Qualitative Observation and Analysis*, Belmont, Cal.: Wadsworth.

Lofland, J. (1976) *Doing Social Life: The Qualitative Study of Human Interaction in Natural Settings*, New York, London: John Wiley & Sons.

MacIntyre, S. (1986) The patterning of health by social position in contemporary Britain: directions for sociological research, *Soc. Sci. Med.*, *23* (4), 393–415.

Marmot, M. and McDowall, M. (1986) Mortality decline and widening social inequalities, *Lancet* Aug., 274–6.

Mullen, P. J. and Reynolds, R. (1978) The Potential of Grounded

Theory for Health Education Research, *Health Education Monog. 6* (3), 280–303.

Neligman, G., Prudham, D., and Steiner, H. (1974) *The Formative Years*, London: Oxford University Press and The Nuffield Trust.

Pahl, J. (1983) The allocation of money and the structuring of inequality within marriage, *Sociological Review 31*, 237–66.

Pill, R. and Stott, N. C. H. (1985) Choice or chance: further evidence on ideas of illness and responsibility for health, *Soc. Sci. Med. 20* (10), 981–91.

Popay, J. (1986) *Patterns of Health and Health Care in Households with Dependent Children*, Progress Report on a Pilot Study, London: Thomas Coram Institute.

Research Unit in Health and Behavioural Change (1988) *Changing the Public Health*, London: John Wiley & Sons, In press.

Rose, G. and Marmot, M. G. (1981) Social class and coronary heart disease, *Brit. Heart J. 45*, 13–19.

Schatzman, L. (1973 *Field Research*, Englewood Cliffs, N.J.: Prentice Hall.

Schutz, A. (1972) *The Phenomenology of the Social World*, London: Heinemann Educational Books.

Stimson, G. and Webb, B. (1975) *Going to See the Doctor*, London: Routledge & Kegan Paul.

Townsend, P. and Davidson, N. (eds) (1982) *The Black Report on Inequalities in Health*, Harmondsworth: Penguin.

Verbrugge, L. M. (1985) Gender and health: an update on hypotheses and evidence, *Journal of Health and Social Behaviour, 26*, 156–82.

Wenzel, E. (1983) Lifestyles and living conditions and their impact on health, in *Lifestyles and Health: European Monographs in Health Education Research*, Copenhagen and Edinburgh: WHO and SHEG No 1.

Whitehead, M. (1987) *The Health Divide: Inequalities in Health in the 1980s*, London: Health Education Council.

World Health Organisation (1986) *Report on the Vienna Dialogue: Health Policy and Health Promotion – Towards a New Conception of Public Health*, Copenhagen: WHO (EURO).

Zola, I. K. (1973) Pathways to the Doctor: From Person to Patient, *Soc. Sci. Med. 7*, 677–89.

13

ROSEMARIE KLESSE AND UTE SONNTAG

HEALTH BEHAVIOUR AND LIFESTYLES OF YOUNG MOTHERS

Background to the study

The project described in this chapter has its roots in many different fields: medical science, epidemiology, sociology, psychology, health and social policy, and the women's movement.

The epidemiological data of the last 20 years in West Germany relating to women's health reveal a number of contradictory findings. For example, on the one hand, women have higher morbidity rates than men but, on the other hand, have lower mortality and a higher life expectancy. This cannot readily be interpreted using quantitative research methods but does lead to important qualitative questions such as: 'Are women ill in a different way to men?' 'What makes women ill?' 'How can women remain healthy?' And, finally, 'What is health if it is not merely the absence of illness?'

The principal hypothesis guiding the study is that so-called health behaviour is influenced by social rather than health factors. Within this formulation, it is necessary to consider both the living conditions conducive to certain lifestyles in women and the way that women are treated in the medical system.

Working-class mothers have been chosen as the subjects of this study for a number of reasons, most of which derive from sociological research. For example, compared with middle- or upper-class women, working-class women have poorer health status and worse health behaviour. They have fewer opportunities for part-time work, are more likely to be unemployed and to be of single status.

158

In addition, as a consequence of the economic crisis, the support for young mothers has declined. In relation to medical care, male physicians may not understand the extent to which women's living conditions affect their health, their health concepts are biased according to the gender of patients and they are not often prepared or able to support their patients in relation to emotional or social problems. Women's changing life perspectives in terms of professional work and education are yet another aspect which has to be considered.

In this project, therefore, we place great emphasis on asking women about their everyday living conditions within the family, about their jobs, their lifestyles and life perspectives since childhood, about their experiences with the official medical system, and about other means they have to obtain information and support when they have problems.

The study is also informed by psychology, since we know that the relation between living conditions and individual health is influenced by intra-psychic factors. It is therefore necessary to consider individual ways of coping – in the long and the short term – with stressful life events and living conditions.

We believe that in order to understand the often ambivalent logic of coping behaviour, research workers must adopt an 'action research' approach and relinquish their 'objective' scientific standpoints and methods. This means that the research worker has to get involved in interaction with the people in the research field. In this interaction, qualitative approaches, subjectivity, participation, equality, a holistic interest and an abandoning of the expert role are all important. These things are a pre-requisite for the development of new and effective health promotion strategies instead of the traditional and ineffective health education methods. Thus, like other community-oriented prevention and health projects, we are using health promotion and lifestyle concepts of the World Health Organisation.

Study design

The study, which began in 1986, is funded by the Federal Ministry for Youth, Family, Women and Health in Bonn.

In the first analytical phase of the study we are conducting qualitative interviews with sixty-five mothers aged between 20 and 35 years. The interviews focus on their health motives and behaviour in relation to their everyday life, their biography and their gender roles. Our long-term interest is to see whether a 'health biography' can be delineated.

Mothers, and especially young mothers, are an important population sub-group because: (a) they are burdened in specific ways and (b) they are thought to be able to change their own behaviour and to have a great influence on their children. We are concentrating on mothers of the lower and middle classes – by which we mean, women without matriculation or tertiary education. We are including mothers with and without paid employment outside the home as well as mothers with and without a partner. All the mothers live in regions which could be defined as 'social problem areas'. This means: high-rise housing, without green spaces, cheap bad flats situated near highways on the periphery of the city of Bremen, where the number of persons receiving unemployment or social-services assistance is above average, where disproportionately high numbers of foreigners and households with many children are found, and where isolation and anonymity of the families and individuals is common.

The sample was obtained, in part, through press releases in local newspapers, but mostly by 'multipliers' such as women in organisations which work with mothers.

At the end of the analytical phase of the study, we intend to discuss our interpretation and evaluation with the women who have been interviewed, the 'multipliers' and our funding organisation. We hope that these discussions will form the basis for the development of a concept of practical health promotion for such mothers.

The second phase of the project is designed to test that health promotion concept in practice. Although we not yet know the results of our interviews nor the health promotion concept to be developed, we already know that there is clearly a great need for health support. Our intention is to implement such support in co-operation with other organisations and initiatives in the form of two health meeting centres within the localities with social problems. Since two health meeting centres have already been established in Bremen as part of the German Cardiovascular Study, we have models and co-operation partners. (The meeting centres are described in the paper, in this volume, by Christel Zenker and Rosemarie Klesse.)

The interviews with mothers. The practical approach to health adopted by the study is demonstrated by the discussion or conversation-guide we use to structure the interviews with the women. In the development of the discussion-guide we tried to operationalise the lifestyle and broader health concepts as well as the biographical approach, to enable us to ask practical questions close to the interviewees life experiences. We try to avoid the interviewees associating the negative aspects of health such as illness and its constituents with our questions. Instead, we try to emphasise the positive implications of the term 'health' and this is developed in discussions with the women by using positive synonyms.

The conversation or discussion-guide which we developed was based on sixteen pre-test interviews. It consists of:

- a definition of health at the beginning and end of the interview
- everyday life in the family and at work
- a personal biography and life history of school and work
- being a woman

Characteristic of open qualitative interviewing is that the conversation is not in the form of a structured questionnaire with 'yes' or 'no' answers. The interviewees are invited to talk frankly about events they consider to be important and to report them as completely as possible; the relevant context, their feelings at the time, their thinking and their explanations. The interviewer thus asks open questions and follows the interviewee in unfolding a theme. The discussion-guide consists of some questions asked as incentives, and also a number of detailed questions, which may sometimes become unnecessary if the interviewees relate such details by themselves in the course of narration.

In order to facilitate the discussion of the implicit and explicit health concept of the individual woman, a defining question in relation to health was asked at the beginning and end of the interview. The definition at the end serves to illuminate possible modification of the interviewees' views which arose during the interview. Thus, at the beginning of the interview, we ask: 'Health has different meanings to everyone. What I am interested in, first, is – personally speaking, what things do you associate with well-being and being healthy?'. At the end of the interview we ask: 'When you think about our conversation once more and the themes of health we discussed: if you were to make a poster about health what would be the important things that should be included for you? What would the poster look like?'

In answer to the defining questions at the beginning, some women expressed a life theme which was particularly important to them. The first rule for the interviewers was to follow the topics that the women suggested. However, if no topics were spontaneously raised the interviewers would suggest 'everyday life' as the next theme. Our focus is on the course of the day; with the different duties within the family; with the work the woman is expected to carry out; the nature of the stress experienced; how this is handled; what she can do for herself; how lack of time influences her feeling of well-being; and what role the social network plays in everyday life especially when problems need to be solved. For instance, we ask: 'And when you think about your everyday life now, are there periods during the course of the day which you experience as burdensome and, secondly, which you enjoy?'. Also: 'And what do you do when you really want to give yourself a treat?'. In addition we talk about orientations in life and ask housewives: 'Would you prefer to have a job?'. Working women are asked: 'Would you prefer to stay at home and not go to work?'; 'How does your role as a mother and housewife affect your job?'; 'What are the effects of your job or of overtime on you and your family?'

We are also interested in everyday life organisation, dealing with time, risk behaviour such as diet, smoking and alcohol, and the social environment and social network. We demonstrate with these questions about women's normal everyday lives that this is, indeed, a worthy subject for research. This is often a surprise for the interviewees.

The next part of the discussion-guide is more personal: the life history and the biography of school and work. Health is a learning process which begins in the family of origin and constitutes itself in the ways in which turning points in life are handled, self-help behaviour, going to professional health experts, personal methods of gaining information, situations of feeling well and wishes in regard to life. We try to trace the salutogenesis, (i.e. personal development in terms of their health biography and in their actual health behaviour). Therefore, we ask, for instance: 'Are there any phrases about health which you remember from your childhood' and 'Remembering your childhood and youth, which important events come to mind concerning health and well-being?' 'How did you come to choose this occupation' and 'If you had wishes in regard to your life, what would they be?'

The final topic 'being a woman' is the most intimate. We tried to develop an atmosphere of trust in the conversation so that by the time we reached this point, we had established an open relationship free from anxiety. We believe that health is connected with the possibility of developing a positive identity as a woman. We talk about how the women see their role, about their experience with menstruation, with sexuality, and with men. For example, we ask: 'Do you remember situations where you liked being a woman very much or where you cursed it?' 'Do you remember what it was like when you had your period for the first time?'

In all parts of the discussion, our aim is to discover the role of norms and values for women in order to understand how this influences their lifestyles in relation to health.

14

AMANDA AMOS AND ANTONIA INESON

BEYOND INDIVIDUAL CHOICE: TOBACCO IN THE PUBLIC HEALTH MOVEMENT

Introduction

In this paper we want to make two arguments, first that the politics of tobacco must be part of the campaign for public health at local, national and international levels; and second, that different types of activity, including research, education and campaigning, can and should support each other in working towards a comprehensive approach to tobacco, or indeed to any other aspect of public health.

If we are concerned to change the public health, it is important to relate activities to the current wider political situation. The present resurgence in interest in public health in the UK is taking place against the background of a government committed to the dismantling of the welfare state, in which assumptions about collective responsibility for health are increasingly threatened. Health campaigners have been attempting to go beyond responding to cuts in health service provision for many years now, both to limit the damage to existing services and to develop ideas – about conceptions of what affects health and about progressive and appropriate services (see for example, Mitchell 1984). The setting up of the Public Health Alliance (Moore 1987), and the action on health being taken by many councils (Moran, 1986) and trade unions (NUPE, 1987) are all part of this.

Tobacco and public health

The polarisation of government and those involved in health campaigning has been reflected in the politics of tobacco in a way which concedes the ground of action to conservative bodies, and which therefore weakens the public health movement. The government's position is that smoking is a question of individual behaviour, which should be countered by single-issue campaigns, through traditionally victim-blaming health education or specific organisations like ASH (Carvel, 1987). Heavy pressure from the medical establishment, mainly the Royal College of Physicians and the British Medical Association (BMA, 1986) has led the government publicly to accept that 'smoking is the biggest single preventable cause of ill-health', but has not succeeded in forcing it to place any significant limits on the freedom of the tobacco industry to produce, promote and sell cigarettes in the UK or worldwide. In this approach, smoking is placed in a hierarchy of preventable risks to health, which usually continues with diet, alcohol consumption, exercise and the risk of contracting AIDS, all of which are seen as matters of individual choice (DHSS, 1976; RCM, 1987). The class and sex distribution of any of these issues is only raised in order to berate working-class people, nurses and northerners about their appalling health behaviour (Carvel, 1987; Lyall, 1987).

So what has the response been from those involved in campaigning for health? In general, with exceptions we will discuss later, it has *not* been a reworking of the politics of tobacco within a public health approach, but rather has often resulted in the rejection of tobacco as a progressive issue. The higher smoking rates of working-class women and men are not recognised as being a success for the tobacco industry, the consequence of lack of government action, and as an integral part of the unequal distribution of resources, power and health. Instead, raising tobacco as an issue has often been seen as an attack on smokers and therefore the working class.

This may partly reflect the strength of the ideology of victim-blaming and individual freedom of choice. It is, after all, commonsense that no one *forces* the smoker to smoke – and confronting commonsense is extremely difficult. The apparent reasonableness of the individualistic approach makes it even more important that the conventional view is challenged at all levels.

For pragmatic reasons, we cannot afford to be entirely opportunistic and work only with certain initiatives, such as those concerned with passive smoking or heart disease, since this is again conceding ground. Instead, activities must form a coherent opposition to the prevailing view that health is fundamentally not a social and political question (Carvel, 1987; Olsen and Tewson, 1987).

Further, it is necessary to go beyond responding to the conventional list of health risks with another list of progressive issues. Little advance is made by replacing concerns such as smoking, diet and exercise with those such as nuclear power and weapons, housing, poverty, unemployment and so on. What is needed is an analysis of how health and disease as a whole are structured under capitalism. The issue does not dictate the politics which surround it. Rather than constructing a unitary hierarchy of health issues, and arguing over whether smoking *or* housing *or* unemployment *or* work hazards *or* the nuclear family, are most important, we need to understand how people's lives are improved or destroyed in a holistic way, always taking account of sex, race, class and other inequalities.

There are many examples of the exclusion of tobacco from serious consideration; one has been the establishment of the Health Promotion Research Trust. This was set up by the tobacco industry in a successful attempt to buy off the government, to prevent any strengthening of the limits on tobacco advertising and sponsorship (Anon., 1985). The British Medical Association (BMA) has been extremely active in campaigning against the Trust, and has advised doctors not to accept money or co-operate with research funded by it. However, people working on drug education, AIDS, health behaviour and work hazards have either accepted funding from the Trust or are considering applying for it. It may be that had the money come from the nuclear industry or a company connected with South Africa, this money would not have been accepted; as it is, the tobacco industry has bought time in which yet another generation of working-class children will become smokers.

The lack of action by the trade union movement is another example, although this is now beginning to change and both individual unions and the Trades Union Council (TUC) have begun to see tobacco as a serious threat to working-class health (NUPE, 1987; ASH/HEC, 1985). The Scottish Trades Union Council (STUC) opposed the establishment of a factory producing Skoal Bandits, tobacco tea-bags, saying that it did not want jobs at such a potential cost to health.

In order to integrate tobacco into public health, it is necessary to move from concentrating on the individual, the smoker, to an examination of the whole chain of production, marketing and consumption of tobacco, the role of the tobacco industry

and governments in this, and the overall effects. This shift has
implications for the type of organisation and action necessary, in
particular the need for international links. This type of analysis
is being developed for other commodities related to health –
for example, for food by the London Food Commission, and
for pharmaceutical drugs. Underlying them all is the recognition
of the ultimate importance of ownership and control. Part of this
would be a more sophisticated understanding of those individuals
and groups who gain from the creation of the unequal distribution
of ill health, within countries and world-wide. Figure 14.1 illustrates some of the areas which would form part of this type of
analysis.

The conclusion, then, is that tobacco does *not* only harm the
smoker, as is often stated, but that it is the product of an industry
and an economic and political system which harms health in a
multitude of ways, which must be understood as a whole if it is to
be changed.

New approaches

The second part of this paper describes some areas where action
has started. Three examples will be used to illustrate some of the
diversity of approaches which are currently being adopted. All have
the long-term aim of improving health and reducing inequalities by
decreasing the level of smoking. They involve a variety of strategies
which have several short-term aims. These include the education
of the public towards a more sophisticated understanding of the
many factors which are involved in the promotion of ill health, and
changing government policy to eliminate all tobacco promotions.

There are now many examples which could have been chosen
from Britain. However, because of restrictions of space, three have
been selected in which the authors have participated. The projects
have involved people and organisations at all levels; individuals,
community and local groups, and national bodies. They illustrate
a key point: that is, how much more effectively these aims can
be achieved through integrating and combining activities which are
often seen as separate and carried out by different people for different reasons. These activities are research, education and lobbying
or campaigning for policy change.

However, in taking an integrated approach, serious consideration needs to be given not only to the field and type of action but
also to, and what is done with, the results.

Women's magazines. Two years ago the BMA launched its anti-
tobacco campaign which aimed to get the government to implement

Related factors	Category	Features	Consequences
diversification e.g. leisure, travel, food companies / dependence upon tobacco companies for finance, fertiliser, market	STRUCTURE OF THE TOBACCO INDUSTRY dominance of multinational companies	based in UK, USA South Africa	
replacement of food by tobacco as a cash crop	PRODUCTION OF TOBACCO largely in the third world	EEC subsidy on tobacco grown in Europe / destruction of forests	
higher tar content for third world markets	MANUFACTURE OF CIGARETTES	in Britain increasingly mechanised	unemployment, especially in areas of existing high unemployment (Glasgow, Belfast)
third world / developed countries	ADVERTISING AND PROMOTION	brand stretching / government controls (and lack of them) in in Britain and elsewhere	
profits returned to countries where industry based	SALES	to children in Britain illegally	

taxation class and sex distribution

the recommendations of previous reports from Royal College of Physicians (BMA, 1986). One of the main recommendations of these reports has been that all tobacco promotions should be banned, and this is linked with the particular area of concern of women and smoking. Women are clearly being targeted by the tobacco industry (Rogers, 1982; Reisman, 1983) and one of the key media which they are using is women's magazines. Women's magazines are read by over half the women in Britain and reach all ages and classes (Jacobson and Amos, 1985). They represent a battleground for anti- and pro-tobacco interests. On the one hand, the tobacco industry targets women through advertising in the magazines; the amount spent on such advertising has increased enormously over the last few years (Jacobson and Amos, 1985). On the other hand, the tobacco industry also recognises the potentially important role that women's magazines can play as sources of information about health, in particular, smoking and women. The very presence of tobacco advertising in magazines is likely to dilute the impact of health information or, as is clear from evidence in the United States, will encourage the magazines themselves to censor out such information from their health coverage (Whelan *et al.*, 1981; Guyan, 1982).

As part of the BMA's campaign, Bobbie Jacobson and one of the authors of this chapter, Amanda Amos, were commissioned to carry out a survey of over 50 women's magazines to investigate their recent coverage of tobacco and smoking and their advertising policies with respect to tobacco. The results from the survey showed that there were numerous breaches of the Voluntary Agreement between the government and the tobacco industry which governs which magazines could accept tobacco advertisements. In particular, the rule which stated that 'media wholly or mainly directed at young people, should not accept tobacco advertisements' was breached (Jacobson and Amos, 1985). Coverage of smoking and health was very low, particularly in those magazines which were most dependent on tobacco advertising revenue.

Having collected the data, the researchers were faced with the question of how the findings could be used to produce changes in policy. The more traditional approach of publishing the results in a medical or scientific journal was rejected in favour of two somewhat different strategies. First the findings were given to the then Director General of the Health Education Council, who expressed his concern to a member of the Board of IPC, the largest publisher of women's magazines in Britain. The second strategy involved the BMA and the Health Education Council jointly producing a booklet *When Smoke Gets in Your Eyes* which summarised the findings in a form designed specifically for media consumption, that is, using appropriate language and quotes from the magazine staff and editors. Both strategies were successful in producing changes in policy.

The Board of IPC changed its advertising policy and banned tobacco advertising from two of their young women's magazines. Perhaps more importantly, considerable debate was generated within IPC as to whether magazine editors felt it was appropriate for them to accept tobacco advertisements. Several pages of their in-house magazine was devoted to this issue (IPC, 1985). The launch of the booklet generated an enormous amount of coverage. Items appeared on BBC and ITV national news and local radio stations on the day of the launch. Articles appeared in national and local newspapers, in medical journals, and magazines such as the *New Statesman*.

One effect of this media coverage was that the public received a considerable amount of information about women's smoking and some of the tactics being deployed by the tobacco industry. The publication of the booklet resulted in a change in the rules governing the placing of tobacco advertisements in women's magazines, despite numerous unfounded criticisms by the tobacco industry. The new voluntary agreement, which came into force a year after publication of the booklet, contained a new clause which further restricted which magazines could accept tobacco advertisements (DHSS/TAC, 1986). The magazines which subsequently stopped taking tobacco advertisements are listed in Table 14.1.

Tobacco promotions and the voluntary agreement. As was mentioned above, there is a voluntary agreement between the British Government and the tobacco industry which aims to control where tobacco promotions appear and what can appear in them. However, whilst previous voluntary agreements have been shown to be subject to widespread breaches there had been little systematic documentation of the scale or nature of such breaches. Therefore, when a new agreement came into force in April 1986, several groups decided to undertake research which aimed to investigate the extent to which the rules in the new agreement were being adhered. Surveys of tobacco promotions which appear on the shop fronts and on hoardings were carried out by two groups, among others. One was a group based in Edinburgh which involved Edinburgh University's Department of Community Medicine, the Lothian Health Education Department and Scottish ASH, and the second was a group of medical students based at the Department of Community

Table 14.1. British Women's Magazines stopped from taking tobacco advertisements by the new Voluntary Agreement on Tobacco/Products' Advertising and Promotion (April 1986)

	Readership* (women over 15)		Readership* (women over 15)
Cosmopolitan	1,815,000	*Company*	701,000
Vogue	1,668,000	*Over 21*	694,000
True Romances	1,077,000	*Ms London*	267,000
Options	1,041,000	*Girl About Town*	217,000
Woman's World	834,000		

* Estimates for readership are from the National Readership Survey (NRS) figures. Jan.–Dec. 1985.

Medicine, St Mary's Medical School in London with support from Paddington and North Kensington Health Education Department.

These two groups looked at the siting of tobacco advertisements, the extent to which they adhered to rules covering health warnings (all tobacco advertisements over 40 square inches should carry a health warning which should be at least 10 per cent of the surface area), and also the extent to which shops displayed warnings about the sales of cigarettes to children. Both studies found that well over half of the shops or advertisements they looked at breached one or more of the rules in the voluntary agreement (Allison *et al.*, 1987; Amos, Robertson and Hillhouse, 1987). The evidence of breaches was submitted to the national Committee for Monitoring Agreements on Tobacco Advertising and Sponsorship (COMATAS) which had been set up by the voluntary agreement (DHSS/TAC, 1986). The St Mary's findings were also presented to their local health authority who, incensed by the scale of the breaches, decided to express their concern directly to the government (Allison *et al.*, 1987). Perhaps most importantly, these and other studies were used to generate media publicity on this issue, in particular the effect that such advertising might play in encouraging children to take up smoking.

The most successful outcome of this so far has been the involvement of the BBC. Initially, Esther Ranzten's popular consumer programme 'That's Life' took up the issue of children and smoking. This was followed by the tea-time health programme 'Go For It' (audience about 7–8 million) which, as a weekly feature, asked members of the public to send them examples of breaches in the rules of the voluntary agreement. They had an enormous response and have submitted the public's evidence directly to the monitoring committee. The tobacco industry responded by putting pressure on Michael Grade, then Controller of BBC1, to take an item out of the programme less than 24 hours before it was due to be screened (Ward, 1987). Of particular interest is the influence that such programmes have had within the BBC. It is highly likely that the approach adopted by this programme, together with the work of John Roberts and Project Smoke Free (Roberts, 1987), was influential in encouraging the BBC to tighten up its rules concerning the broadcast of tobacco-sponsored events, such as snooker.

Thus, research findings were used both to lobby for policy change and to increase public awareness. Enormous publicity was given to the failure of the tobacco industry to abide by the rules of the voluntary agreement by the 'Go For It' and Esther Rantzen programmes. The impact of these programmes should not be underestimated. For example, when carrying out a follow-up study on tobacco advertising in Edinburgh and a small study in Stoke-on-Trent, surveyors were stopped several times by children and asked if they were involved in the Esther Rantzen or 'Go For It' programmes. The participation of medical students in the St Mary's survey also has important implications for innovative ways of training health workers. The students left the environs of the medical school and went out into the community to study the factors influencing health at first hand and as a result became involved in taking action themselves. They were able to see what are often regarded as individually determined behaviours within their wider social, political and economic context.

TREES. The last example has a different starting point, not research, but lobbying for policy change. Over the last few years in Britain there has been an emergence of several new lobbying groups, such as AGHAST (Action Group to Halt Advertising and Sponsorship by Tobacco) and COUGHIN (Campaign on the Use of Graffiti for Health in Neighbourhoods). The group we wish to concentrate on is TREES (Those Resisting an Early End from Smoking) which was set up in part to counter the activities of FOREST (Freedom Organisation for the Right to Enjoy Smoking Tobacco) which is funded by the tobacco industry. By creatively picketing tobacco-sponsored events, the aim of TREES is to obtain media coverage which shows up the hypocrisy of the tobacco industry's tactics. It bases many of its tactics on those of the Australian group MOPUP (Movement Opposing the Promotion of Unhealthy Products) (Chapman, 1980).

Members of TREES are drawn mostly from health professions but also include other interested individuals, smokers and non-smokers. Over its 2-year history, it has picketed events throughout the country including the Benson and Hedges Cricket Final at Lords, Rothmans Snooker in Cardiff, Embassy Snooker in Sheffield, the Benson and Hedges Photography Exhibition at the Stills Gallery in Edinburgh and Hamilton's Gallery in London, and John Player Special sponsored ballet at the Festival Hall, London. There have also been several one-off media events such as the delivery of a coffin containing cigarette butts and animal bones to the head-quarters of Imperial Tobacco in London. The hearse in which the coffin arrived was covered with the message 'Think Black', with the JPS logo on a black coffin. These, and other events, have created considerable media interest and coverage. TREES activities have been covered by local, national and foreign newspapers, national and local television and radio, and have even been mentioned on NBC news in America.

TREES has directly lobbied policy makers, for example, the then Minister for the Arts when entering the JPS sponsored Portrait Exhibition at the National Portrait Gallery in London. Picketing of the Embassy sponsored snooker at the Crucible in Sheffield was followed by the City Council changing its policy on accepting tobacco sponsored events. The City Council decided as part of its anti-tobacco policy not to accept any new contracts for tobacco sponsored events on council property.

Examples of TREES activities have been used in a wide variety of educational settings to encourage school children, students and other health workers to explore the wider issues involved in the tobacco debate. Medical students at several universities throughout Britain, in particular Edinburgh and Southampton, regularly have teaching on the activities of TREES and the politics of tobacco. TREES also gives talks to other health workers such as nurses and health education officers during their in-service training. A news-letter is produced by TREES for members in Britain and it is also sent to organisations in other countries such as to the Consumer Association of Penang in Malaysia, thereby sharing information about strategies, successes, failures and lessons learnt.

The impact of these diverse activities is obviously difficult to assess. However, it is clear that TREES is now accepted by the media as a legitimate organisation whose activities and media coverage are of considerable concern to the tobacco industry. For example, when Radio London recently produced a half-hour programme based around TREES activities, the Tobacco Advisory

Council complained to the Director General of the BBC. This resulted in the radio producer being demoted. It was claimed that the BBC was showing 'bias' and the issue was reported in the industry magazines *Tobacco* (Anon, 1987; Adams, 1987) and *Tobacco Reporter* (Stone, 1987), although without mentioning TREES, possibly a compliment to TREES' campaigning methods.

Conclusion

The examples, described in this paper illustrate how a public health approach to tobacco is being developed in Britain which includes action at all the levels advocated by the Ottawa Charter on Health Promotion (WHO *et al.*, 1986).

Thus as well as focusing on the need to develop personal skills, which is often the only aspect of smoking prevention covered by the more traditional victim-blaming type of health education, these activities go considerably further by lobbying for healthy public policy, that is, a ban on all tobacco promotions. This will create supportive environments, particularly for children who will be less likely to be influenced by glamorous images of smoking, especially those generated by tobacco-sponsored sports (Ledwith 1984). Community action is encouraged and strengthened by the involvement of the media, which can focus individual and community concerns on particular issues and direct these concerns to those involved in policy development within the government. Finally, the involvement of health workers in organisations such as TREES, and teaching about TREES activities in in-service training, helps to broaden their understanding not only about tobacco but also the need to reorientate the health service away from a primarily curative approach to a service that is truly health promoting.

References

Adams. (1987) Who at the BBC monitors the bias? *Tobacco*, February, 37.

Allison, M., *et al.* (1987) Tobacco advertising – the facts, Paper presented at the 31st Annual Scientific Meeting of the Society for Social Medicine, September, Dublin.

Amos, A., Robertson, G., Hillhouse, A. (1987) Tobacco advertising and children: widespread breaches of the voluntary agreement, *Health Education Research*, 2, 207–14.

Anon. (1987) BBC producer censured, *Tobacco*, January, 3.

Anon. (1985) Taking money from the devil, *British Medical Journal* 291, 1743–4.

Action on Smoking and Health/Health Education and Health (1985)
    Action On Smoking at Work. London: ASH.
British Medical Association (1986) *Smoking Out the Barons*, Chi-
    chester: John Wiley & Sons.
Carvel, J. (1987) Commons debate on health promotion, *Lancet*, 1037–8.
Chapman, S. (1980) A David and Goliath story: tobacco advertising and
    self regulation in Australia, *British Medical Journal*, *281*, 1187–90.
Department of Health and Social Security (1976) *Prevention and Health
    – Everybody's Business*, London: HMSO.
Department of Health and Social Security/Tobacco Advisory Council
    (1986) *Voluntary Agreement on Tobacco Products' Advertising and
    Promotion and Health Warnings*, London: TAC.
Guyan, J. (1982) Do publications avoid anti-cigarette stories to protect
    ad dollars? *Wall Street Journal*, November, 22.
IPC (1985) IPC rules on tobacco ads. IPC News, May/June, 1–5.
Jacobson, B. and Amos, A. (1985) *Smoke Gets in Your Eyes*, London:
    BMA/HEC.
Ledwith, F. (1984) Does tobacco sports sponsorship on television act
    as advertising to children? *Health Education Journal*, *43*, 85–8.
Lyall, J. (1987) Nurses' lifestyle attacked, *Health Service Journal*, 13
    November, 1305.
Mitchell, J. (1984) *What is To Be Done About Illness and Health?*,
    Harmondsworth: Penguin.
Moore, W. (1987) Building a public health alliance, *Health Service
    Journal*, 23 July, 842–3.
Moran, G. (1986) Radical health promotion – a role for local authori-
    ties?, in Rodmell, S and Watt, A. (eds) *The Politics of Health
    Education*, London: Routledge & Kegan Paul.
National Union of Public Employees (1987) Equality in health – a
    strategy for change, London: NUPE.
Olsen, N. D. L. and Tewson, N. (1987) Government to take health
    seriously?, *British Medical Journal*, *295*, 941–2.
Radical Community Medicine (1987) *AIDS and Oppression*, 31
    Autumn.
Reisman, E. (1983) Look to the ladies, *Tobacco*, March 17–19.
Roberts, J. (1987) *Name of the Game: Cigarettes on BBC TV*, Man-
    chester: Project Smoke-Free.
Rogers, D. (1982) Editorial. *Tobacco Reporter*, February.
Stone, M. (1987) Has balance gone from the BBC? *Tobacco Reporter*,
    February 6.
Ward, S. (1987) Bias fear halts BBC smoking film, *The Independent*,
    15 May.
Whelan, E. M., Sheridan, M. J., Meister, K. A., *et al.* (1981) Analysis of
    coverage of tobacco hazards in women's magazines, *Journal of Public
    Health Policy*, *2*, 28.
WHO/Health and Welfare Canada/Canadian Public Health Association
    (1986) *Ottawa Charter for Health Promotion*, Copenhagen: WHO.

Information and the Public Health

15

IRVING ROOTMAN

USE OF A NATIONAL SURVEY TO CHANGE THE PUBLIC HEALTH: CANADA'S HEALTH PROMOTION SURVEY

Research can be a powerful tool for changing the public health. This paper looks at an attempt to use research for this purpose in the hope that others may learn from the experience. In particular, it describes efforts to use a national health promotion survey to promote health in Canada.

The survey in question is Canada's Health Promotion Survey which was carried out in June 1985 by Statistics Canada (Canada's national statistical agency) on behalf of the Health Promotion Directorate of Health and Welfare Canada. Approximately 1,000 respondents per province or territory were interviewed to determine their health knowledge, attitudes, beliefs, intentions, practices and status as well as some of the factors contributing to health practices and status including the influence of family and friends and environmental conditions. In all jurisdictions with the exception of the Northwest Territories, respondents were selected by random digit dialling and interviewed by telephone. In the Northwest Territories, because of the lack of telephones as well as cultural considerations, respondents were selected to be representative of the three major ethnic groups there and interviewed face-to-face. Overall, the response rate was 81 per cent. The survey was restricted to Canadians over the age of 14 who were not living in institutions.

The purposes of the survey were to provide information to be used for: the planning, development and evaluation of the Health Promotion Directorate programme (the federal government body responsible for health promotion efforts at the national level in

178

Canada); planning, development and evaluation of other health promotion programmes in Canada; and for communication to the public. This paper describes how the information resulting from the survey have been used to achieve these purposes as well as to achieve some unanticipated purposes consistent with an attempt to improve the health of Canadians.

As suggested by our primary purpose (use for planning and development of Health Promotion Directorate program) we have provided relevant information from the survey to staff of our own Directorate. In fact, we even involved a number of them in analysis of the data. A good example of this would be the analysis of data on smoking of young women which we carried out in collaboration with one of the program staff of our Tobacco Unit. That Unit had become increasingly concerned about the elevated smoking rates of young women in Canada and wondered whether anything could be done about it.

A multiple discriminant analysis was done using Health Promotion Survey data and it was found that the best predictor of smoking among young Canadian women was the number of friends they had who smoked and the second best was the belief that 'smoking was a good way to stay slim'.

This information was fed into the Federal-Provincial committee responsible for the National Program on Smoking in Canada and they are presently developing new initiatives based on this new information. Although we have not as yet used data from this survey to evaluate the federal health promotion programme, we are about to undergo major evaluation of the total program in which data from the Health Promotion Survey compared to earlier survey data will be used.

The survey has, however. already begun to satisfy the second purpose (planning, development and evaluation of other Health Promotion programs in Canada). This has been facilitated by the fact that we made the data available to provinces at exactly the same time as we received them. As a result, most provinces have carried out their own analyses and many have produced their own reports along with recommendations for provincial action.

One of the things that makes the data particularly valuable to provinces is the design of a survey which includes provincially representative samples. This allows each province to compare themselves with the country as a whole on a wide range of health attitudes and practices.

Figure 15.1 illustrates one such comparison. It shows the percentage reporting use of seat-belts in Canada, the province of

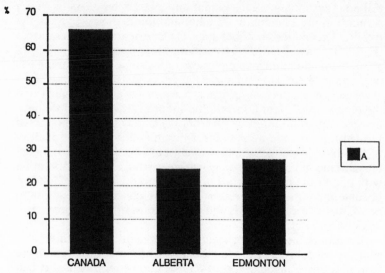

Figure 15.1. Self-reported seat-belt use in Canada, Alberta and Edmonton, 1985 health promotion survey.

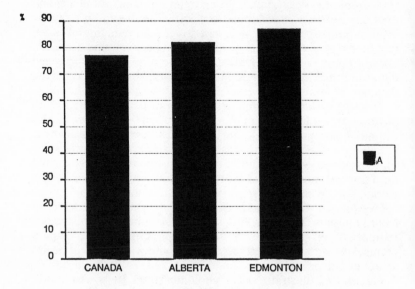

Figure 15.2. Smoke detectors in the home in Canada, Alberta and Edmonton, 1985.

Alberta and the city of Edmonton (which was the only city surveyed at the same time as the national survey took place). As can be seen, Albertans and Edmontonians are much less likely than other Canadians to use seat-belts – a finding which is probably accountable for by the fact that at the time of survey Alberta was one of the only provinces without compulsory seat-belt legislation.

On the other hand, however, as indicated in Figure 15.2, Albertans and Edmontonians are more likely to have smoke detectors in the home than residents of other provinces. Thus, as was the case for every province, Albertans performed better than other Canadians on some health practices and attitudes and worse on some others.

Such provincial profiles have so far proved to be very helpful to provinces in allocating their health promotion efforts.

With regard to the last purpose (to inform the general public), we have done this in a number of ways. For example, we used Press Conferences and releases when the first report from the survey was released. But more important was the press coverage when we engaged in a series of Federal-Provincial exchanges which usually took the form of workshops whose participants were invited by the provincial government hosts. The press was invited to attend each exchange and there were a series of television, radio and newspaper interviews of both Federal and Provincial officials.

They tended to emphasise how provinces stood in relation to the rest of the country but also emphasised issues relevant to health promotion such as the need to reduce inequities in health and increase prevention. Thus, it is clear that the survey accomplished its intended purposes to some degree at least. But perhaps, more important, it has accomplished a number of unintended purposes as well. For example, giving tapes to provinces had the side benefit of enhancing collaboration between Federal and Provincial governments in Canada. Similarly, the exchanges have built working relations between the federal government, provincial governments, local governments, voluntary organizations and community people working in the field of health promotion in Canada. In addition, the survey has accomplished other things that were unanticipated but which, in the end, could have a major impact on the public health in our country. Specifically, it has challenged some of the ideas of people in the field of health promotion and it has contributed to the development of national health promotion policy in Canada.

The main vehicle for release of findings so far is The Active Health Report (Health and Welfare Canada, 1987). In contrast

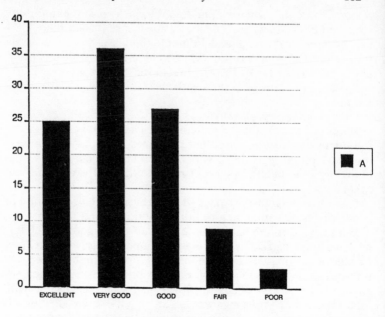

A

Question: "In general, compared to other persons your age, would you say your health is excellent, very good, good, fair or poor?"

Figure 15.3. Self-rated health among Canadians, 1985.

to most reports on surveys, it is not hard to read nor is it filled with tables. It is, rather, a report designed for health promotion practitioners with as much weight, if not more, given to interpretation as to data. Its main purpose in fact is to raise issues and challenges for the field of health promotion and each chapter ends with an 'issues' and 'challenges' section. To draw an example from the first chapter of the report, as can be seen from Figure 15.3, the majority of Canadians rate their health rather well (61 per cent as very good or better) but who is it that rates their health as excellent?

It is clear from Figure 15.4 that many people who rate their health as 'excellent' practice what many health promoters might consider poor health habits. From the point of view of health promotion, it raises the question of whether we should accept their perceptions as valid and build instead on their desire to remain healthy or should we try to counsel them that they are not as healthy as they seem to think they are? If so, can we teach them to rate their health more accurately?

The Active Health Report does not try to answer these questions

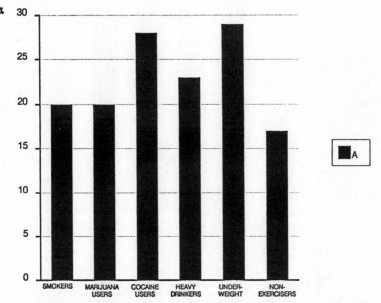

Figure 15.4. Proportions of Canadians rating health as 'excellent' by health practices, 1985.

but challenges health promotion practitioners to discuss them and try and find answers. And they have indeed provoked considerable discussion in the field as have the questions raised in other chapters of the report.

With regard to the contribution of the report to policy development, as an unplanned but fortuitous coincidence, while we were analysing data from the survey, our Minister decided that he would like to release a major policy paper on Health Promotion at the Ottawa Conference on Health Promotion in 1986.

A number of those who were working on the survey data were assigned to work on the policy paper. The end product was a paper entitled *Achieving Health For All: A Framework For Health Promotion* (Epp, 1986).

It would probably be fair to say that this document could have been produced without benefit of the survey, but it would also be fair to say that many of the ideas generated in developing the Active Health Report have enriched the document.

In addition, it is quite clear that data from the survey provide some added empirical support for the policy. For example, one of

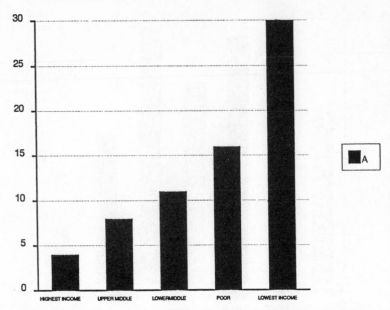

Figure 15.5. Proportion of 25–64-year-old Canadians rating health as fair or poor, 1985.

the challenges for health promotion is 'Reducing Inequities'. Figures from the Health Promotion Survey (Figure 15.5) shows that in addition to a relationship between income and 'so-called' objective measures of health, there is also a strong relationship between income and a subjective measure. This holds for other measures of socio-economic status including education and unemployment.

Similarly, the survey provides some additional evidence of the potential of 'mutual aid' – one of the three mechanisms identified for addressing the challenges for health promotion. The survey suggests that there is a strong relationship between our own practices and those of our friends. For example, in Canada, if our friends smoke we are seven times more likely to smoke than if our friends don't. Similarly, if our friends drink heavily we are nine times more likely to do so ourselves.

This holds for spouses too. If our spouse uses marijuana we are forty-two times more likely to do so than if they do not. If our spouse uses tranquillizers we are five times more likely to. The relationship holds for positive as well as negative practices. If our spouse or friends exercise, we are twice as likely to do so than if

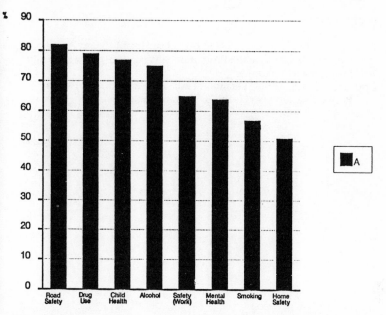

Figure 15.6. Proportion of Canadians considering government action to be 'very important' by issue, 1985.

they do not. More dramatically, if our friends don't use marijuana our chances of doing so are one in a hundred. We don't know if these relationships are causal, but they are certainly important for health promotion. At the very least they suggest the need to learn how to use friendship networks to improve health.

Finally, Figure 15.6 indicates support for one of three strategies identified in the Minister's paper, namely, Healthy Public Policy. As can be seen, there is enormous support for government action on a wide range of health promotion issues, most of which need intersectoral collaboration.

To conclude, it should be clear that Canada's health promotion survey has been used constructively to try to improve the public health. Whether these efforts will in fact result in such improvements remains to be seen but, based on our experience to date, we are optimistic that they will in fact help us to achieve 'health for all' Canadians.

References

Health & Welfare Canada (1987) The Active Health Report Perspectives on Canada's Health Promotion Survey, 1985, Ottawa: Health Promotion Directorate.

Epp, J. (1986) Achieving Health For All: A Framework for Health Promotion, Ottawa: Health & Welfare Canada.

16

BERNARD PISSARO

A PUBLIC HEALTH INFORMATION DATABASE
AVAILABLE TO ALL: THE RAMIS NETWORK

Introduction

RAMIS is a public health information database developed in 1984 by a number of public health teams in France willing to give access to relevant documentation to those who need it: the various partners who play a role in public health may need this facility whether they be health professionals, decision-makers, elected representatives, association or union representatives or lay people. A greater knowledge of processes, methodologies, parameters and experiments of public health will allow all, at their respective levels of responsibility, to bring relevance to their actions. In addition, the development of an active and efficient approach to information will contribute greatly to health promotion and reduce some of the high costs incurred by poor information. Most of the founding teams in the project already had more-or-less developed 'libraries' and felt the need to computerise them for better control of their resources, thus rationalising common ownership of material.

This is the context in which RAMIS was born. Its general direction is public health, which comprises many fields, such as community health, health promotion and health policy. Because of the multidisciplinary nature of public health there is a need for a variety of approaches and points of view which take into account a whole range of associated topics such as epidemiology, socio-anthropology, economics, environment and geography.

The content and remit of RAMIS

In France there are over fifteen documentation centres specialising in health information. The documents acquired and generated
by these centres can be borrowed, read or sent for; the total
number of documents held by the different centres is around 16,000
and comprises books and brochures, journals, bibliographies, sets
of slides, films, cassettes and records, videocassettes and teaching
material. About 30 per cent of these are common to several centres,
but each centre owns and acquires material to suit its own specific
requirements and orientations.

To make better use of this mountain of material, information on
available resources needed to be developed and access to the system
facilitated. This meant combining: (1) a document index: a list
of all the centres in the Network; (2) an information system:
the RAMIS Database; and (3) a communications system:
access through a terminal (e.g. MINITEL) to this database. It
was therefore necessary to compile a directory of all the 'libraries'
which keep information on public health. This directory will shortly
be available on MINITEL. A computerised index of people and
institutions specialising in public health is also being prepared;
and an electronic mail system to facilitate communication between
the various partners is being set up.

RAMIS is therefore to become a 'health memory', by acting
as guardian of the database, by allowing access to documents and
therefore knowledge, by being an organised directory which grows
and adapts constantly. In its finality it will be accessible to all.
RAMIS will give access to references of all books, journals and
other non-published literature, as well as audio-visual material.
This material has been collected by the network since 1st January,
1986 and produced by the network's participants. There will be
8,000 new entries in the database each year. This will allow the
user to undertake their own research in their own order of priority.
However, knowing of a document's existence is not enough; the
user needs to obtain it.

The database is like a giant reservoir where the location of each
document will be identified:

> if it is common to all the centres, the names of fifteen centres
> will be given;
> if it is kept in only one or a few centres, these will be named;
> if it is not kept by any centre, it will not be found in the
> database.

The requested document will be obtainable through the network's participants or a lending centre and soon through MINI-TEL. In addition, the directory listing all documents centres will enable the user to identify the nearest centre.

Selection of documents and updating of information

All health information for dissemination to the public will be included. Very specialised documents or those for use by CNRS (Centre National des Recherches Scientifiques) will not be included; however, possibilities of obtaining access to CNRS networks, particularly FRANCIS, are being studied. All literature produced by the Ministry of Health should also as a rule be included. In the field of health information, all documents produced in the past decade will gradually be added to the database.

Centres will be responsible for notifying and updating the datbase of each new acquisition. Prior to doing this, the centres will be able to make sure that notification has not already been made and if it has, the centres will be required to inform the database that they too have the document; this can be done by keying in the centre's nine-digit code. During the updating process, each notification will go into the sub-directory and all indexes will be automatically updated.

Access to a database

One can access a database in different ways:
(1) By querying 'on line': for this, a professional terminal compatible with the file server is needed. The user will be billed for the telephone connection and for the call itself, the charge varying with the duration of the call. On-line querying will shortly be available to all from the beginning of 1988, through MINITEL.
(2) By contacting a documents centre, whether a network participant or not, which in turn will query its own database and the whole network.

To assist the user, the network participants have set up a thesaurus of 3,500 key search words. The user can look for acceptable synonyms, for broader terms or, on the contrary, for more specific terms. The thesaurus can be updated to suit needs without delay. There are two advantages to this approach:
The system is able to interpret the user's own words;
The chances of getting the required information are increased.

The parameters

It was no easy task to set up such a database. Several parameters had to be considered:
1. *The documents.* (a) The documents were scattered among

regions and institutions and processing and acquisition procedures were not rationalised.

(b) The volume of data: 8,000 new entries a year with a goal of a database containing up to 100,000 entries.

(c) The sheer variety of the material.

(d) The diversity of fields relevant to public health: all relevant topics are exhaustively covered, with special emphasis on two topics: health promotion and health in the work-place.

(e) The different levels of needs to cater for: those of health centres, hospitals, consumers associations, city and town councils, ministries, etc.

(f) The different users: all health-related staff and health services partners, (i.e. users) elected representatives, association representatives, company management teams, researchers, etc.

(g) Several millions of health services customers are potentially interested, even if they are only very gradually becoming aware of the importance of having access to documentation.

2. *The structure.* (a) Each team had to be encouraged to improve its ability to disseminate information on its own resources, by making optimum use of the network.

(b) The preparation of documents had to be rationalised, by encouraging the sharing of processing tasks.

(c) The work and experiments carried out regionally had to be integrated into the set-up.

(d) Existing equipment in regional centres had to be made use of by developing diversified regional initiatives thus achieving optimum decentralisation: making the database accessible to the user's own MINITEL.

(e) The financing at national level of co-ordination efforts, technical developments and personnel training programmes. Co-operation had to be encouraged between all centres and partners for a non-lucrative purpose. The aim was to ensure coherence of the system.

Establishing the database

1. In 1984 a feasibility procedure was carried out which focused on: cost effectiveness, legal considerations, technological considerations, and the needs of those the project aimed to serve had to be assessed.

A census was carried out of those keeping documentation; this formed the basis for the first directory and matched the numerous initiatives, particularly from the ORS (Regional Health Bureaus).

2. In 1985/86 the first full-scale trials were carried out. The thesaurus was developed and assessed, giving the network its own operating language, a vital support if the network is to have a long life expectancy.

The pilot project was refined by the document centres participating in the network, taking into account the recommendations emanating from the feasibility study. The possibility of transfering the developed programs to other network's participants was looked into and assessed, thus allowing direct access to the finalised mode of operation.

The directory was computerised and an initial list of 750 addresses can already be looked up through MINITEL or through a computer terminal.

Following a technical assessment, SUNIST (National University Technical and Scientific Information Server) was chosen as file server.

3. 1986/87: The network opened to the public. Despite major financial problems, the network increased its capabilities, utilities were developed and co-ordination with the RHESUS Network of CNRS is entering a concrete and practical phase; it will be possible to interrogate on line the index of 5,000 references with summaries, available from now on from the participating centres. It is expected that on line ordering will be in place by the next stage.

The advantages of health information

The database will give access to documents as they are published which describe, analyse, comment on, criticise, dissect and explore from all possible angles, the subject of health in France.

This information is essential, as was pointed out earlier, to those who need to be '*au fait*' with the orientations and operation of the health services, to those who have to participate in the decision-making process with regard to health: whether it be at the local, or regional or national level; whether or not they belong to the medical profession; and whether or not they are still in training. This information is essential because it encourages the user to study, discuss or reflect on the subject and is therefore a condition of the evolution and adaptation of the health services to the needs of the public; it also facilitates the best possible use of services in the field of health promotion and also in hospitals or among the medical profession. It is not enough to want to improve the performance of the services without the means to do so; it is of paramount importance to improve the information and training for medical personnel, the public and elected representatives.

Some prospective studies have shown that continuous staff training schemes will soon take up to 10 per cent to 15 per cent of a worker's working week; part of this training is individual and made possible by the development of new information technology. Medical staff should not be exempt from this, as training is based on information. For this reason it is essential to bring wanted information to peoples' homes and to facilitate access to documents in every possible way.

Database for the lay public. The database was developed to answer health needs. Therefore, as part of the indexed resources, documents which have been produced especially for use by non-professionals or existing ones which are sufficiently clear and easy to understand will be included. It may be that such documents from the database can be extracted and made available as a separate category to the lay public directly through MINITEL. Nevertheless, the whole database should still be open to the public for information.

The unsolved question of financing the scheme with regard to the user's contribution remains. One solution put forward was to vary the size of the fee according to the type of user. For example, school pupils are potentially important users but should not expected to be able to pay for the service. While accepting that the costs of thinking up and developing the database will be covered in the main by public monies, it remains that local bodies will have to cover the fees charged to the user. Giving people the means to inform themselves should be an integral part of the educational strategy.

Cost effectiveness. The database will make a number of savings possible, as well as providing a better service for users and generating income. First, the tasks of analysing and indexing documents will be shared, thus allowing the network's archivists to do other tasks such as dealing with and informing the public, helping with research, managing and organising audiovisual libraries. Secondly, a major part of document research, which used to be cumbersome and time-consuming, will now be carried out in minutes.

From now on it will be possible to edit automatically and catalogue (by subject, field, etc.) documents which were not generated by the network's centres. It will also be possible to research documents and edit them to suit the user's needs. This, therefore, represents an increase in the quality of service. It is impossible, of course, to quantify the improvement in the quality of information at the disposal of the user. However, this can be assessed systematically.

An efficient database can be sold, as a whole with all its contents, or in different parts, such as its software, languages, etc. It generates income each time it is made use of and each time documents are sold.

The future. A long-term stance is essential. The data will be transferred on to computers with a large storing capacity. It will therefore become easily available to the user from the work place at low cost. The audiovisual libraries will release materials which cannot be transferred on to computers without corruption of quality or content. All the computerised data can be accessed and read from machines with screens. The machines are technologically sophisticated enough to enable users to browse through texts, pictures and sounds at high speed; it will also enable them to find their way to information by using everyday language (written or spoken).

To bring about this information revolution, data need to be stored, and software and lists of key search words need to be assembled. The latter will be necessary until the time when the use of natural language is a reality. Health establishments must also be equipped.

17

HEATHER ROBERTS AND PAMELA GILLIES

PREVENTION INDICATORS FOR HEALTH PROMOTION

Introduction

The evaluation of health promotion activities is crucial to the planning and co-ordination of effort and to the effective deployment of dwindling health-related resources. Such evaluation has, however, rarely assumed a prominent position in the integrity of the development of health promotion programmes (Noack and Abelin, 1987). In addition, few of the attempts to measure health promotion have been comprehensive, covering the wide range of individual behaviours, organisational change and individual or group interactions which could possibly be affected (Kar and Berkanovic, 1987). It could be argued, however, that this has less to do with reluctance to tackle the existing methodological and other difficulties which such an all-embracing approach would require, but more to do with the urgent need to gain an indication of the relative effectiveness of at least some aspects of programmes at a time when health service resources are under considerable constraint.

Catford (1983) has commented on the need to develop cheap, simple community surveys to measure health-related behaviour in populations to determine the effectiveness of health-promotion activities. This simplistic approach is justifiable on the grounds that healthy behaviours have been shown to be directly related to mortality and physical health status (Catford and Nutbeam, 1987; Hamburg *et al.*, 1982; Berkman and Breslow, 1983; Reed, 1983) and to mental well-being (Kar, 1984; Chrisman and Kleinnan, 1983).

194

To date, a number of studies have been carried out which attempt to measure health-related behaviour. Table 17.1 illustrates six of these surveys and highlights the lack of any definitive method for collecting self-reported data about health.

In the search for the application of the most appropriate and efficient means of collecting information of this type, opportunities for increasing the public's awareness of health issues and the priming for health behaviour and possibly also environmental or service changes, could be explored and developed. Previous studies have made no attempt to use the method of data collection itself to engage public interest or commitment, or to feed back information to individuals, groups, 'communities' and institutions.

This paper describes a pilot study which aimed to develop methods of collecting and distributing data about health with a view to stimulating awareness about health issues and encouraging a 'readiness' for health promotion activity.

The process of survey methodology, in itself, was therefore deemed to be as important as the ability of the method to establish baseline data for the evaluation of programmes in terms of the possible impact of health-promotion activities upon individuals' behaviour, knowledge and attitudes and upon the prevailing environment.

Methods

Sample. Three quota samples of 240 persons were compiled from general practitioners' lists, attenders at doctors' surgeries and community network sources.

Two types of areas were chosen to offer contrasting types of samples for the pilot study. One was a predominantly working-class area, the other middle class. Census Small Area Statistics were used to identify the areas (OPCS, 1982). Occupations were classified using the Registrar General's Classification by Occupation (OPCS, 1980). The working-class areas used in the study were the mining towns of Bolsover and Shirebrook in Derbyshire. Geographically close, the towns are similar demographically, with manual, working-class populations of 58 per cent and 62 per cent respectively, from total populations of approximately 11,000.

Data collection. (i) *Questionnaire.* Data were collected by a self-completed questionnaire. Bearing in mind the findings of the Black Report (Townsend and Davidson, 1982), and the Health Divide (Whitehead, 1987), it was recognised that the lower the social class, the higher the risk of disease related to health behaviour

Table 17.1. Six examples of methods of collecting self-reported data to measure health-related behaviour

Survey report	Method of self-reported data collection		Selection of sample	No. of respondents
	Interview	Self-completed questionnaire		
1. A study of health beliefs, attitudes and behaviour among working class mothers. Pill, R, and Stott, N. C. H. (1983)	×		age/sex register	204
2. An Apple a Day. Butler, J. R. (1987)		×	random	2,110
3. Colchester Borough Health Survey M.V.A. Consultancy (1986)		×	random	2,760
4. Health and Lifestyle, Health Promotion Trust. Stenney, R. (1987)	×	×	random	9,000
5. Protocol and questionnaire, Welsh Heart Programme. Directorate (1985)	×	×	random	22,000
6. Wigan Health Survey. O'Donnell, P. (1986)	×		random	486

and the higher the likelihood of reading and writing difficulties (Roberts, 1986). Possibly 10 per cent of the population may be illiterate or semi-literate (Levine, 1986). Consequently, great care was taken to ensure that the self-administered questionnaire was readable, relevant, easy to complete and easy to return.

Questions included those related to key health behaviours identified in the Korner Report (HMSO, 1984): smoking, alcohol, diet and exercise. In addition, questions about participation in health-screening programmes, perceptions about the power people think they have over their own health and knowledge about AIDS were also included.

(ii) *Administration*. Questionnaires were delivered by three different, non-overlapping methods, based on doctors' or health centres' catchment areas. At this stage of the study the aim was simply to see if any of these methods of delivery gained a response from the public. These methods were:

(a) By post, to every tenth adult male and every tenth adult female on a general practitioner's list.

(b) By general practitioner's receptionist to patients attending surgery and their adult family members.

(c) By community networks.

All questionnaires were accompanied by a self-addressed, pre-paid envelope for return. The community networks method was a more novel approach to delivering questionnaires and needs further explanation. Community networks involved using key individuals within existing structures, (e.g. health visitors), in a given 'community' (defined as the catchment area of a general practice) to act as agents to deliver questionnaires to people they knew personally.

(iii) *Feedback of information*. The questionnaire offered respondents the opportunity to receive selected leaflets on health issues and a 'local community' summary of the health behaviour reported in the questionnaires on request. This innovative form of feedback was perceived to be crucial to harnessing potential interest in individual and group health promotion activity.

Results

The main objective of the pilot study was to generate a reliable instrument for measuring health behaviour and to record the level of response obtained from each method of questionnaire delivery. Responses are shown in Figure 17.1. As quota samples were used, the absolute difference in response by method may be attributable to the type (bias) of samples obtained. Figure 17.1 shows that all methods received response without a reminder process. The response from the networking method in both middle-class and working-class areas was better than that from the postal questionnaire, but not as good as the response to the delivery by receptionist. The pilot study established that the community network method of distribution did operate and did generate response. Analysis of the demand for feedback about health (Figure 17.2) shows that there were as many, if not more, people from working-class areas as there were from middle-class areas, who wanted the information offered about health and a local summary of the study findings.

For example, 40 per cent of respondents from the working-class area compared to 33 per cent of respondents from the middle class area requested information about healthy eating, whilst 22 per cent of respondents from each area wanted information about heart disease, and 13 per cent more respondents from the working-class than the middle class area wanted information about local health behaviours.

Discussion

It has been argued that the will of individuals and communities is the key to achieving improved health (Mahler, 1977). If this is true, then it seems that the only way forward is to strive actively to create conditions wherein the will to change can be generated and can flourish. Continuing to criticise those who fail to adopt healthy life-styles despite health promotion campaigns is perhaps both harsh and unproductive (Gillies *et al.*, 1987). The challenge for health promotion is to create realistic possibilities for change, particularly for those who cannot see how, at the moment, they may create these possibilities for themselves, thereby stimulating the will to improve health, both individually and collectively.

This pilot study has demonstrated that it is possible to introduce a survey methodology, using existing community networks, in which the *process* designed to promote change, is as, if not more, important than the *outcome*. The methodology, therefore, offers health promotion a tool which not only helps to identify conditions which mitigate against health, but which, if used sensitively, may also enable individuals and the community, together with health professionals, to work towards change.

The following example, using data from the pilot study, suggests ways in which change may be effected. The survey showed that, of respondents who lived in an area where a large chemical factory was sited, and who also felt that pollution made their health worse,

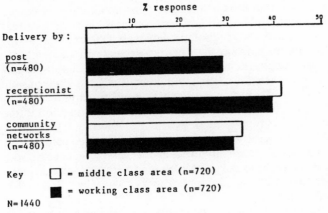

Figure 17.1. Responses to survey by delivery method by social class of area.

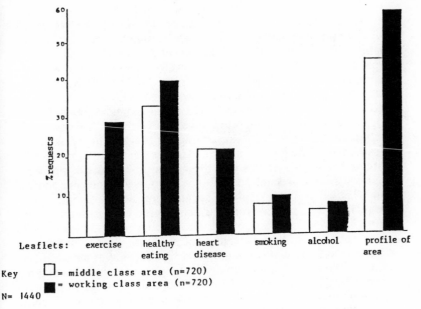

Figure 17.2. Percentages of requests for information leaflets by social class of area.

85 per cent said that they could do nothing about the pollution to which they were exposed. There are two possible ways forward: first, to use feedback to prompt debate within existing groups about the findings from the survey; second, to draw people together to discuss their collective concerns and support legitimate action – such as inviting comment from those responsible for the pollution, creating a pressure group to explore ways of reducing pollution or, using local media, to draw attention to the problem.

As agents for creating opportunities for change, feedback of information to all those involved in the survey in concert with community networking may be identified with the radical survey approach proposed by, amongst others, Roy Carr-Hill (1984) who comments that:

> Since social change can be carried out only by people, measures and statistical activities should be organised on the human level and organised around possibilities for change.

The intrinsic value of community networking lies in its process rather than its outcome. It should be recognised that data obtained by this process is unlikely to be a representative sample of a population. Indeed, one of the attractions of the method lies in the fact that the survey may be directed towards specific groups within a community, for example, the unemployed or the elderly. Information produced via community networks must therefore be seen as complementary (but not additive) to information obtained by a postal survey from a representative sample drawn from the same 'community', using local doctors' age/sex registers for a sampling framework. The groups of particular concern to health promotion are working-class groups who are known to be more at risk from certain diseases related to health behaviours and the environment in which they live (Health Education Authority, undated) and less likely to conform to the advice offered by health-promotion activities (Pill and Stott, 1987). Such groups seem to be less likely to respond to surveys (Quigley and Williams, 1986). Preliminary findings suggest that community networking may be a particularly appropriate survey methodology for these groups since, of the three types of questionnaire delivery methods used in the pilot study, community networking obtained the highest proportional initial response rate from working class adults, although the working class was under-represented in all methods of questionnaire distribution.

One of the aims of the main study, of which this was the pilot, will be to document change, not only of individuals' behaviour and knowledge, but also at organisational, environmental and community levels. Essentially, the pilot study has shown that a survey committed to feedback of information and using community networking does offer the potential to act as a priming agent for change in a way that is not an integral part of other survey methodologies. The process of surveying using both community networking and statistically acceptable survey methodology means that health promotion has available to it a flexible, action research tool which will help to identify priorities for health promotion programmes and provide a method of evaluating health promotion. It may also lay the foundations for future work in which communities are prompted to engage in the process of change, thereby helping themselves to create local conditions in which the will to improve health may be generated.

References

Berkman, L. F. and Breslow, L. (1983) *Health and ways of living*. Oxford: Oxford University Press.

Butler, J. R. (1987) *An Apple a Day*, Health Services Research Unit, University of Kent at Canterbury.

Carr-Hill, R. A. (1984) The principal choice of social indicators, Economic Paper 371, University of York.

Catford, J. C. (1983). Positive health indicators – towards a new information base for health promotion, *Community Medicine 5*, 125–32.

Catford, J. and Nutbeam, D. (1987) Breathing life into Wales, *Health Trends*, May.

Chrisman, N. J. and Kleinnan (1983) Population health care, social networks and cultural meanings. in Mechanic, D. (ed.) *Handbook of Health, Health Care and the Health Profession*. New York: Free Press.

Gillies, P. A., Madeley, R. J. and Power, L. (1987) Smoking cessation during pregnancy – a controlled trial of the impact of new technology and friendly encouragement, Paper presented at the 6th World Conference on Smoking and Health, Tokyo.

Hamburg, D. *et al*. (1982). *Health Behaviour Frontiers of Research in Bio-behavioural Science*, Washington: Institute of Medicine, National Academy of Sciences.

Health Education Authority (no date given), *Health Education: Guide to Healthy Eating*.

Kar, S. B. and Berkanovic, E. (1987) Indicators of behaviour conducive to health promotion, in Abelin, Brezezinski and Carstairs (eds), *Measurement in Health Promotion and Protection*, Copenhagen: WHO.

Kar, S. B. (1984) Psychological environment: a health promotion model, *International Quarterly of Community Health Education*, *4*, 311–41.

Korner, E. (1984) 4th Report of the Steering Group on Health Service Information, London: HMSO.

Levine, K. (1986) *The Social Context of Literacy*, Routledge & Kegan Paul.

Mahler, H. (1977) Problems of medical affluence, *WHO Chronicle*, *31*, 8–13.

MVA Consultancy (1986) Colchester Borough Health Survey.

Noack, H. and Abelin, T. (1987) Conceptual and methodological aspects of measurement in health and health promotion, in Abelin, Brezezinski and Carstairs (eds), *Measurement in Health Promotion and Protection*, Copenhagen: WHO.

O'Donnell, P. for Wigan Health Education Department (1987) Wigan Health Survey.

Office of Population Censuses and Surveys (1982) *Small Area Statistics*, London: HMSO.

Office of Population Censuses and Surveys (1980) *Registrar General's Classification of Occupation*, London: HMSO.

Pill, R. M. and Stott, N. C. H. (1983) Report to Health Education Council.

Pill, R. M. and Stott, N. C. H. (1987) The stereotyping of 'working class fatalism' and the challenge for primary care health promotion, *Health Education Research*, June 2, Pt.2, 105–14.

Quigley, C. and Williams, J. (1986) Stockport Health Survey. Stockport: Stockport Health Authority.

Reed, W. L. (1983) Physical health status as a consequence of health practices, *Journal of Community Health*, *8*, 217–28.

Roberts, H. R. (1986) Literature for Parent Education. M.Phil. Thesis, University of Nottingham.

Stepney, R. (1987) Health and Lifestyle Survey, Health Promotion Research Trust, Assets House, 17 Elverton St, London.

Townsend, P. and Davidson, N. (1982) *The Black Report on Inequalities* in Health, Harmondsworth: Penguin.

18

SARAH CURTIS AND SOPHIE HYNDMAN

THE NEED FOR CHANGE IN INFORMATION, ORGANISATION AND RESOURCES: A STUDY OF HOUSING DAMPNESS AND RESPIRATORY ILLNESS

Housing dampness is a problem which affects large numbers of people in Britain. It is estimated that 2 million homes suffer from severe dampness and a further 2.5 million suffer to a lesser extent (Building Research Establishment, 1986). In one of the larger household surveys on this subject, Hunt and Gidman (1982) found that of 1,000 homes, 46 per cent reported a damp problem, and 20 per cent of these had mould growth.

The majority of studies investigating health in damp homes do indicate a detrimental effect on health, especially respiratory health (Martin *et al.*, 1987; Strachan and Elton, 1986; Burr *et al.*, 1981; Holma and Kjaer, 1980; Rasmussen *et al.*, 1978; Todd, 1984; Holts Tenants Group, 1979; Bedale, 1983). Both the extent of dampness and its possible relationship to respiratory health imply that housing in the UK is in need of urgent and considerable improvement, and that failure to address this problem is resulting in poor health for a large number of people. Thus, dampness appears to be a widespread problem, and the possibility that it has health implications makes it a concern for public health.

This paper considers dampness in council housing and its relationship to respiratory morbidity in parts of the London Borough of Tower Hamlets. The relationship between health and housing is a particularly good example of the complexity of public health issues, and the difficulty of implementing effective policies to bring about change. The paper concludes with some comments about the applications of this type of research and on the need for better local co-ordination of statutory and voluntary organisations to achieve changes which will be necessary to ameliorate the types of problem we observed in the survey.

Background to the study

Tower Hamlets is located in London's East End, and can be shown on the basis of many criteria to be severely socially and economically deprived. For example, the amenities available within the homes are on average poorer than for British households as a whole. The level of overcrowding in Tower Hamlets is also comparatively high, with 10 per cent of households having more than one person per room (the highest figure for inner London). The Under-Privileged Areas Indicator, a composite social indicator, which is often used to assess relative levels of urban deprivation relevant to health need, has a value for Tower Hamlets of +55, showing it to be one of the most deprived areas in the country according to this measure (Irving and Rice, 1984).

The health status of the population in Tower Hamlets is also relatively poor compared with other parts of the country. The overall standardised mortality rate is comparatively high for London, and the borough has mortality rates due to respiratory disease and tuberculosis which are among the highest in the country (OPCS, 1981). Survey data also indicate that compared with Redbridge, a suburban borough in East London, people in Tower Hamlets are more likely to report symptoms of respiratory disease such as catarrh, sore throat, cough and breathlessness (Curtis, 1983; Curtis, 1986).

Thus both housing dampness and respiratory illness are a more serious problem in Tower Hamlets than elsewhere in the country. This paper reports on the preliminary results from a household survey in one part of Tower Hamlets which investigated housing dampness, mould growth and respiratory health. Aggregated population data have severe limitations as a basis for epidemiological analysis of the relationship between housing conditions and health, and there is a lack of precise information on factors such as subclinical, or untreated respiratory problems, dampness and mould growth in housing. It was clear that data were required at the level of individuals, and that this would need to be collected using community survey techniques.

A local survey of housing and respiratory health

The study was informed by other studies which have investigated the problem of housing conditions and health (Holma and Kjaer,

1980; Rasmussen *et al.* 1978; Hunt *et al.*, 1986; Strachan and Elton, 1986). The study controlled some of the variables which would effect the relationships of interest. A limited number of housing blocks were selected for study, of a similar structural design, and in the same area, and where the resident families were of similar socio-economic status and from distinct cultural groups. Other studies had encountered problems because they relied on self-reported data on health and housing conditions, and we were particularly interested to compare 'objective' measurement with the more 'subjective' reports of respondents.

Method. The survey was conducted in a part of Tower Hamlets where housing conditions and health were both relatively poor. The study area was selected mainly on the basis of a screening questionnaire which was sent to all the Tenants' Associations in Tower Hamlets to identify estates with particular problems with dampness. Two estates were selected for investigation. All the flats in these estates were covered by the survey. Data were collected on 204 households representing 54.6 per cent of the total number of dwellings. The information reported here cannot necessarily be generalised to Tower Hamlets as a whole, and the results we have obtained reflect the circumstances of families in an area where the conditions give particular cause for concern. In the 204 households examined, a total of 761 residents were covered by the survey.

One respondent, where possible the female head of household, was selected from each household, who also provided information by proxy on other members of the family. At each dwelling, an interview was carried out with the informant concerning family characteristics, reported housing conditions and reported respiratory morbidity. At the same time, measurements were made with a Burkard personal air sampler, to assess mould growth and atmospheric spore concentrations, and where possible, a sample of mould was taken and grown for identification. Temperature readings were also taken, and relative humidity was measured using a whirling hygrometer. As an 'objective' measure of respiratory health, a mini Wright peak-flow meter was used for the measurement of the lung function of any family members present. Thus the survey included reported and mechanically measured conditions in the household.

Results. (1) *Housing.* In 95 per cent of the homes, the accommodation was rented from the council, and 90 per cent were maisonettes and flats of a similar design. The percentages of households with problems are described in Table 18.1. The presence of damp rooms was significantly related to cold rooms and whether

Table 18.1. Proportion of households reporting various housing characteristics

Housing characteristic	Percentage of households with the characteristic
Central heating	8.0
Inadequate heating	74.5
Heating 'too dear'	45.6
Adequate ventilation	81.0
Draughts	40.0
Inadequate insulation	73.5
Cold rooms	88.0
Damp rooms	72.5
Mould growth	57.0
Unusable rooms	20.0
Dissatisfaction with home	52.0
Likelihood of improving conditions	32.0

or not there was central heating. Housing type also seemed to be a significant factor in the prevalence of damp; flats and maisonettes at the ends of blocks appearing to be particularly prone to dampness.

We were also interested to see how objective measures of damp, cold and mould related to the respondent's perception of damp and cold. In homes where damp rooms were reported, relative humidities were significantly higher (mean 64.4 per cent) than in homes where no damp rooms were reported (mean of 55.5 per cent). The level of relative humidity considered critical for the growth mould is 70 per cent. In homes where damp was perceived to be a problem 64 per cent had relative humidities below this threshold, and the proportion with relative humidity above this level was 36 per cent. In homes where dampness was not perceived to be a problem, only 17 per cent had relative humidities above the critical threshold. Overall, there was a statistically significant association between perceived and measured dampness. Households reporting cold rooms had an average temperature of 12.9°C, about 2°C below those not reporting cold rooms (average 25.2°C degrees). Households reporting mouldy rooms had a mean fungal spore count of 28,959/m³ against those not reporting any mould problems who had fungal spore counts with an average of 9,589/m³, a significant difference. Fungal spore counts also showed significant differences depending on the presence or absence of damp rooms in the home. The average fungal spore count in homes, with damp

Table 18.2. Proportions of the respondents reporting respiratory morbidity

Types of complaint	Percentage of respondent with the complaint
Bronchitis	11.0
Chesty colds	51.4
Asthma	4.0
Depression	12.4
Cough during the night	23.0
Cough during the day	18.0
Wheezing	14.0
Breathlessness	15.0
Blocked-up nose	25.0
During the last two months	
Aches and pains	30.0
Headache	30.0
Tiredness	26.0
Vomiting	7.0
Diarrhoea	7.4
Trouble with nerves	14.0

was $25,995/m^3$ compared with $9,393/m^3$ in homes with no damp rooms. In three homes fungal spore counts of over $100,000/m^3$ were recorded. The highest spore count was $482.477/m^3$.

(2) *Health.* Table 18.2 shows for the 761 people covered by the survey, the percentages of the respondents reported to have various health complaints.

Peak flow was found to be significantly lower for respondents reporting one or more of the following symptoms: nocturnal or diurnal cough, blocked-up nose, wheezing and breathlessness. Those reporting symptoms had a mean peak flow of 78.5 compared with 90.8 for those free from all of these symptoms. Those reporting bronchitis, chesty colds, asthma or tuberculosis (past or present) had significantly lower mean peak flows (80) than those free from these health problems (86.1). Both of these relationships persisted when demographic variables (sex and age group) were taken into account, as shown by contingency tables and analysis of variance. This implies that the reported morbidity data are related to the objective peak-flow data.

A stepwise multiple regression was conducted to investigate the possible relationships between dampness in the home and respiratory health (Table 18.3). The objective peak-flow measure was

Table 18.3. Stepwise regression model showing the significance of various facto peakflow (dependent variable = peakflow)

Independent variables (significant in equation)	Standardised beta coefficient	T-value	Significance of T	Adjus R-squa
Age	−0.49553	−8.704	0.0000	0.257
Smoker	−0.19543	−3.453	0.0007	0.288
Damp rooms	−0.12973	−2.303	0.0222	0.302
Independent variables (not significant in equation)				
Sex	0.03626	0.636	0.5253	
Humidity	0.09075	1.579	0.1158	
Fungal spore count	−0.07849	−1.399	0.1632	
Temperature	−0.01586	−0.272	0.7861	

* Adjusted R-squared shows the progressive total variation in peakflow accou for as each independent variable is added to the equation. The change in R-sq when a particular independent variable is entered into the equation shows the additional amount of variation in peakflow explained by the independent varia

used as the dependent variable representing respiratory health. The independent variables tested were: age, sex, whether the respondent smoked and the presence or absence of dampness as reported by the respondent. Taking into account age and smoking behaviour, which were significantly associated with peak flow, a significant association was also found to exist between reduced peak flow and dampness in the home. However, the actual predictive value of the association was small using this kind of analysis. The objective measures of dampness (spore counts, relative humidity) were entered into the regression model but they did not show a significant association with peak flow.

Discussion: the validity of subjective and objective measures. Both the objective and subjective techniques employed have their strengths and weaknesses. The efficiency of the objective measures has to be weighed up against their suitability as tools in a community survey when equipment needs to be portable and measurements have to be conducted in the home of the respondent. The ease of employing subjective measures of health and housing conditions should be balanced against their reliability and it may be that conclusions drawn from subjective measures carry more weight if their reliability can somehow be assessed in terms of objective indicators.

The results seemed to indicate a relationship between self-reported housing conditions and respiratory function, but a less clear association between health and objective measures of domestic environment. One possible reason for the less-clear relationship found when using the objective measurements could be the over-reporting of housing problems by respondents with poorer respiratory health. It is possible, however, that the objective measurements themselves are causing some of the confusion. For example, in the cases of temperature and humidity, these were 'spot' measurements taken in only one room and as such may not have reflected the conditions typical of the home as a whole. The environment in each room would depend on its structural design (e.g. number of external walls) and the use made of it. Conditions in each room might vary over time according to the level of occupancy and the activities carried on there (e.g. cooking, bathing, etc.).

A final consideration is that the peak-flow indicator itself can be quite an erratic measure of respiratory health, its value depending to some extent on the aptitude of the person being assessed

Some general conclusions can be reached from the preliminary analysis of this survey. There appears to be a significant relationship between reported measures of respiratory health and those measured objectively using a peak-flow meter. There also seems to be significant associations between reported housing conditions and measured temperatures, relative humidities and fungal spore concentrations. This would suggest that associations found between housing conditions and health in studies that have used only self-reported techniques may well be reliable sources of data and should not be dismissed lighly. We have found a possible link between housing dampness and respiratory health using an objective measure of health and self-reported housing conditions.

Approaches to achieving change

While poor housing conditions, including dampness, are clearly a matter of concern throughout the country, which would justify better policies and intervention at the national scale it appears that, in the short term, the most effective means to improve housing is likely to be based on local initiatives. We conclude by considering what are the ways in which research findings of the type reported here may be used for this purpose, and what other strategies may be successful.

The work reported here has been done with reference to local groups, and the results will be made available to them.

Well-researched evidence of levels of housing problems and morbidity may strengthen the arm of local residents' associations, especially tenants, who are struggling to improve their housing. In some areas, for example in Balloon Wood, Nottingham (Balloon Wood, 1981), and on one of the estates covered by this survey (CCAG and SHAPRS, 1985), the strength of local action combined with professional help (for example, from independent surveyors) has provided a convincing and well-documented argument for change in their local areas. The importance of local law centres should also be recognised in their successful attempts to help individual tenants and, more recently, groups of tenants from a whole block (Ormandy, 1986). It could be that a closer collaboration between tenants' groups and professional bodies, such as these, can produce change on a local basis. However, some estates may lack the coherence to produce concerted action on their own behalf, and it is in these communities that the poorest housing conditions are often to be found. It may be necessary to provide residents in this type of area with expert assistance to stimulate self-help activity.

Any tenant action, however well co-ordinated, will come upon problems when facing badly co-ordinated and ill-funded local bureaucracies. The problem of council housing conditions detrimental to health is a clear example of a public health issue which crosses the boundaries of responsibilities of local authorities and health authorities, and requires co-ordinated effort to effect change. While health authorities may feel the impact of poor housing conditions, which give rise to morbidity and demands on the health service, they have little power to affect the quality of housing for patients. In the case of council tenants, they may exert pressure for rehousing of tenants on medical grounds, but in an area like Tower Hamlets, with many priority cases on the waiting lists, this will have only a limited effect. Furthermore, this is a reactive measure to the impact of poor housing on health, rather than a preventative approach which might take effect before ill health occurs.

At the same time, local authorities may lack the motivation to act. Environmental health officers, themselves officers of local authorities, are in a particularly difficult position in trying to improve housing conditions for council tenants. Having been divested of most of their other health-related functions in the 1974 local government reorganisation, local authorities have, in general, not been active in questions relating to health. However, the recent growth in the numbers of local authorities with health committees and working parties is beginning to redress this situation, and to extend the environmental health role into a more wide-ranging health promotional activity (Fryer, 1987). The encouragement by the Association of Metropolitan Authorities for this type of initiative is now being echoed at a more moderate level by the Association of County Councils (Smith, 1987). This type of body within local authorities seems likely at least to engender awareness of public health issues in local authorities, and may help to promote a more responsive attitude to health-related issues.

In order to make real progress with the problem of housing and health in an area as challenging as Tower Hamlets, it seems that concerted action of local authorities and District Health Authorities is necessary. This seems a very appropriate area for joint funding, which until recently has been mainly spent on initiatives for provision of domiciliary welfare services. However, some Joint Consultative Committees are now realising that joint funding may help to tackle some of the health-related housing problems in deprived inner-city areas. In Tower Hamlets, for example, there is a proposal to find joint funding for a community public-health worker to act as a facilitator, in order to stimulate local action to combat problems of domestic and outdoor environmental quality.

Certainly the quality of housing is an issue which is likely to remain prominent in the revived debate concerning public health. It is seen as a matter of importance by the public as well as researchers and health and welfare professionals. Community surveys in Tower Hamlets (e.g. Curtis, 1983; Lauglo, 1982) have shown that the problems of housing and the local environment are viewed by local people as serious problems, more important than questions concerning lack of money, illness, or quality of local health services. The Tower Hamlets Health Inquiry (1987) has included among its recommendations the need to improve living conditions for people in the area, and the Tower Hamlets Strategy Group is a working group with members representing local residents, community interest groups, health and welfare professions and academics, which is trying to help to realise some of these recommendations. This is, perhaps, an example of the type of coalition which will be increasingly necessary to take up the challenge of changing the public health in the future.

References

Balloon Wood (1981) What the experts say about Balloon Wood.

Bedale, C. (1983) Health and housing project, Manchester Road. *Comm. Med. 14*, Summer ed, 12–14.

Building Research Establishment (1986) Remedies for condensation and mould in traditional housing (video).

Burr, M. L., St Ledger, A. S., Yarnell, J. W. G., (1981) Wheezing, dampness and coal fires, *Comm. Med.*, *5*, 205–9.

CCAG and SHAPRS (1985) Chicksand Community Action Group and Spitalfields Housing and Planning Rights Service. *Chicksand: Coming out of the cold?*, A report on the need for heating on the Chicksand Estate.

Curtis, S. (1983) Intra-Urban Variations in the Health and Health Care. The comparative need for Health Care Survey of Tower Hamlets.

Curtis, S. (1986) Self reported morbidity in London and Manchester. Intra-urban and inter-urban variations, *Social Indicators Research 19*, 255–72.

Fryer, P. (1987) Oxford's aim of health for all, *Health Service Journal 5*, March 1987, 274–5.

Holma, B. & G. Kjaer (1980) Alcohol, housing and smoking in relation to respiratory disease, *Environment Research*, *21*, 126–42.

Holts Tenants' Group (1979) *Families at risk. Dampness and ill-health on Holts Estate.*

Hunt, D. R. G. and Gidman, M. I. (1982) A national field survey of house temperatures, *Building and Environment*, *17*, 102–24.

Hunt, S. M., Martin, C. J., Platt, S. D. (1986) Housing and health in a deprived area of Edinburgh. Unhealthy housing, a diagnosis. IEHO conference, Warwick University, 14–16 December.

Irving, D. and Rice, P. (1984) Information for health services planning from the 1981 Census. Kings Fund Centre, London.

Lauglo, M. and Malpern, P. (1984) The Spitalfields Health Survey Tower Hamlets, Department of Community Medicine, London.

Martin, C. J., Platt, S. D., Hunt, S. M. (1987) Housing conditions and ill-health, *BMJ. 294*, 1125–7.

OPCS (1981) *Area Mortality 1969–73*, Series DS4, London: HMSO.

Ormandy, D. (1986) Togetherness wins, *Roof*, September/October, 29.

Rasmussen, F. V., Borchenius, L., Winslow, J. B. and Oster-Gaard, E. R. (1978) Associations between housing conditions, smoking habits and ventilatory function in men with clean jobs, *Scand. J. Resp. Dis.*, *59*, 264–76.

Smith, J. (1987) Detecting a health care revival, *Health Service Journal*, 23 April.

Strachan, D. P. and Elton, R. A. (1986) Relationship between respiratory morbidity in children and the home environment, *Family Practice*, *13*, 137–42.

Todd, S. (1984) Danger, a health risk, *Comm. Action 64*, Feb/March
     27–9.
Tower Hamlets Health Campaign (1986) Health and housing survey
     preliminary results.
Tower Hamlets Health Enquiry Report (1987) Copies obtainable from
     Community Health Journal, 23 New Road, London E1.

19

GRAHAM BICKLER AND LESLEY MORRISON

THE PUBLIC HEALTH RESPONSE TO THE CHERNOBYL DISASTER

Introduction

On April 26th 1986, a nuclear power reactor at Chernobyl exploded and radioactive material was released into the atmosphere. People in the Ukraine were evacuated for a radius of up to 100 miles. The response in other countries varied. The DHSS sent a circular to all Medical Officers for Environmental Health (MOEH) on May 2nd, set up a phone enquiry service on May 6th, sent a letter to all Port Health Authorities on May 13th and one to all Regional Medical Officers on June 27th about foreign travel. The National Radiological Protection Board (NRPB) issued daily press releases from May 2nd. Official advice in the UK included washing fresh vegetables well and not drinking rain water. Sales of lamb from hilly areas in North Wales and Cumbria where contaminated rain had fallen was controlled. There is disagreement about the level of radioactivity which constitutes a public health risk and about the level at which action should be taken.

Despite the vast amount of media coverage and public anxiety, the Department of Community Medicine in Hackney only received one enquiry about the local situation. As community physicians we found it difficult to know how to respond to it and we were also unclear as to what steps we might or should have taken ourselves.

Survey

We decided to carry out a national survey of community physicians in order to find out how many enquiries they had received

214

Table 19.1. Response rate

	Number of Questionnaires sent	Maximum possible number of replies	Numbers of districts replying	Numbers of responses used
England	191	188	175	169
Wales	9	9	9	9
Scotland	15	15	11	10
	215	212	195 (92%)	188 (89%)

in the wake of the Chernobyl disaster and what their response had been to it, to examine their perceptions of the national public health response and to identify improvements that could be made in the system.

A short questionnaire was sent to all 215 District Medical Officers (DMOs) or their equivalent in England, Wales and Scotland in July 1986. They were asked to complete it themselves or refer it to the most appropriate person. Non-responders were sent a follow-up letter one month later.

Results. Replies were received from 195 districts (or equivalents). The data from some were amalgamated locally by the MOEH, reducing the maximum possible number of replies to 212. Three replies were incomplete and one was returned too late to analyse, giving a response rate of 89 per cent (Table 19.1).

DMOs were asked how many enquiries they or their department received up to the end of May 1986 from the public, the media, or health workers, about the implications of, or appropriate response to, the threat of low-level radiation. Fewer than six enquiries were received by 60 per cent of DMOs, and more than ten were received by only 20 per cent (Table 19.2).

The 160 respondents (DMOs) who received enquiries were asked what responses they made to them. Of these, 87 per cent gave reassurance, 79 per cent gave advice and 50 per cent referred the enquiries to another agency. The most frequently used agencies (and the number of respondents who used them) were the National Radiological Protection Board (26), medical physics departments (11), DHSS (7), Ministry of Agriculture, Fisheries and Food (7) and the Foreign Office (7). More than ten other agencies were mentioned.

The DMOs were asked what other action, either as a result

Table 19.2. Number of enquiries received by DMOs

Number of enquiries	Number of DMOs	(%)
Not answered	1	0.5
0	27	14
1–5	86	46
6–10	37	20
11–20	17	9
20	20	11
	188	100

of the enquiries, or independent of them, they had taken. Of the total, 52 per cent attempted to acquire information about local levels of radiation and their possible health consequences, 15 per cent used the local media to issue a statement, 55 per cent liaised with other health workers and 18 per cent took some other action. This ranged from one DMO who wrote to the Chief Medical Officer to complain about administrative chaos and one who contacted the local emergency planning officers, to an unsuccessful attempt by one to use a geiger counter. Those who attempted to acquire information about local levels of radiation (97) did so from twenty agencies, of which the most frequently used were: NRPB (19), DHSS (17), MAFF (16), medical physics departments (15), environmental health departments (11) and water authorities (10). This demonstrates the difficulties that community physicians faced in getting clear policy and information. This is confirmed by the even larger number of organisations to whom ninety–seven of the DMOs turned when they themselves were trying to find out about local radiation levels. Several DMOs commented that the press was the most reliable source of information!

The fact that only 2 per cent of the respondents expressed satisfaction and 44 per cent expressed dissatisfaction with the national response to the disaster can only be an indictment of the system. Furthermore, criticisms were made more frequently by those respondents who attempted to discover local radiation levels and by those who received most enquiries (Table 19.3), suggesting that it was the attempt to deal with the situation locally that led to dissatisfaction.

The main theme which emerged from the criticisms was a lack of

Table 19.3. Percentage of DMOs critical of national response by number of enquiries received and by attempt to discover local radiation levels

Number of enquiries	% Critical of national response (n)	
0	(27)	18
1–5	(86)	43
6–10	(37)	51
11–20	(17)	53
20	(20)	60
Did attempt to discover local levels	(97)	50
Did not attempt to discover local levels	(84)	38

confidence in official information in terms of its quality and availability. Typical comments were: 'Advice was out of date before it arrived'; 'Telex and letter from DHSS too late and too brief to be of any use'; 'The Government response to this situation and its possible effects in this country was too little and too late'; 'A shambles generally – diverse bodies giving diverse advice'; 'It was a blind leading the blind situation'. Several respondents referred to the implications for disaster planning in the UK: 'What will happen when the bomb drops?'; 'What would we have done with a melt down?'. All this led some DMOs to be grateful that there was little attempt by the public to gain information from them: 'Fortunately, public concern locally was minimal'. The DHSS acknowledged these difficulties. An official said: 'There can be no doubt that all community physicians should have been better provided with information'.

There are several ways in which these improvements could be achieved. Some of the more constructive suggestions were: the establishment of a Communicable Disease Surveillance Centre type body which would deal with environmental pollution and toxicology; the appointment of a minister with a specific responsibility for the co–ordination of information and advice in similar future situations; and the development of a CEEFAX/PRESTEL type information system for DMOs/MOsEH. One respondent suggested that this incident might stimulate the Faculty of Community Medicine to take the lead in the co-ordination of research and policy-making in this area.

The lack of good public health information that this survey has highlighted demonstrates the urgent need for the development of effective information systems before such a disaster is repeated.

Subsequent events

On June 20th 1987 the Prime Minister replied to a question in the House of Commons about what action the government had taken since Chernobyl. She said that contingency plans were being prepared and, in the event of a similar episode, the Department of Environment would be the lead department. A network of monitoring stations based on existing facilities and an efficient communication system was being developed. She referred to a national response plan for nuclear incidents overseas which would organise treatment and monitoring arrangements.

The plans were put out for consultation to local authorities via the Institute of Environmental Health Officers, by the National Radiological Protection Board. It was circulated on July 14th 1987 with the final date for receipt of responses on July 24 1987. One particular criticism of it was that it concentrated on gathering information through the monitoring system but failed to describe clearly how the information would be disseminated and made accessible.

The Prime Minister also referred to plans to cope with a nuclear accident inside the UK. These would be based on the Health and Safety Executive's publication *Emergency Plans for Civil Nuclear Installations*. This document was first published in 1982. It was produced primarily for the benefit of those concerned with the preparation and implementation of emergency plans. However, in its introduction it also stated: 'publication of this information should help to reassure members of the public, especially those who live or work near nuclear plants, that detailed and well-rehearsed plans exist for their protection in the unlikely event of an emergency'. This emphasis on reassurance was continued later in the document: 'An accident at a nuclear plant . . . is highly unlikely to pose a significant threat to public safety or require actions to protect the public which are different from those required for other civil emergencies. The most likely outcome of any accident at a nuclear plant is that no one would be hurt at all'.

The DHSS has also produced a planning document about civil nuclear incidents in the UK. It is currently out for consultation inside the government but it is expected to be sent out to Health Authorities within the next few weeks and definitely by the end of the year. This will be the first official communication about planning received by Health Authorities from the DHSS since Chernobyl. The previous one, *Health Services Arrangements for Dealing with Major Accidents*, was published in 1985 (HC (85)24) and tended to emphasise the role of Health Authorities in providing reassurance: 'Following a reference accident the levels of radiation dose or contamination of people outside the site would be very unlikely to cause harm to health and would require little action by the Health Service apart from reassurance'.

After the Chernobyl experience, we must hope that the final documents are useful and realistic. What has been seen so far does not inspire confidence. We can be optimistic and trust that such plans will never be needed, but the possibility of further major civil nuclear disasters abroad or in the UK demands serious planning.

Acknowledgements. We would like to thank Dr Ken Grant and Dr Sian Griffiths for their help and encouragement.

References

Dunster, J. (1986) *New Scientist*, How we reacted to Chernobyl. 5th June, 62–3.

Lambert, B. E. (1986) *The Consequences of the Russian Nuclear Incident*, Department of Radiation Biology, Medical College of St Bartholemew's Hospital.

**Professional Behaviour:
New Roles and Structures**

20

MICHEL O'NEILL

THE POLITICAL DIMENSION OF
HEALTH PROMOTION WORK

This paper does not present the final results of research. Based on the author's fifteen years of involvement as a practitioner, researcher, consultant, militant and teacher in the fields of community health and health promotion, it discusses a much forgotten issue: the political dimension of health promotion programmes and policies. This discussion will be conducted in three sections. In the first, a few definitions are provided as well as an appraisal of the current state of the health promotion field. In the second section, the lack of interest of health promotion workers in the political dimension of their job will be presented, along with some tentative explanations of this phenomenon and some of its consequences. Finally, the third section will provide information on the preliminary work conducted to develop tools for the integration, by health promotion workers, of the political dimension of life in their daily work; it will also reflect on constraints occurring when, as an academic person, one wants to gain access to the kind of applied work required to help health-promotion professionals to increase their political skills.

The political dimension of health promotion

By political dimension, we refer to the existence in any group of human beings of power relationships that influence (in a very significant, although not exclusive, manner) the behaviour of individuals, groups, communities or nations (O'Neill, 1987b). By power relationships is meant, as most political scientists would agree, the capacity of certain groups or individuals to constrain other groups or individuals to behave in certain ways. Health promotion, in agreement with concepts recently revamped under the leadership of the World Health Organisation European Office (WHO, 1986; Kickbusch, 1986; Charter, 1986), can be considered as:

> Any action, incentive or coercion, to influence (populations, specific groups, legislators, governments, professionals, grassroots organizations, etc.) and aimed at changing lifestyles or the environment in which these lifestyles have developed. (O'Neill, 1987a, 15; free translation)

The political dimension of social life. To add a little to these definitions, it should first be pointed out that constraint may be enforced on people by various means. The most obvious ones are physical, be they applied individually or socially by organisations like armies or police corps, or by less legitimised ones like the Mafia or other underground groups. However, it is no less obvious that psychological constraints may sometimes be used as effectively as physical ones to prompt people to behave in certain ways.

As a second word of caution, it should be emphasised that the political determinants of human behaviour are not necessarily the most important ones; depending upon the situation, biological, psychological, social, cultural or other sets of factors may be central to understand why individuals or collectivities act in a certain manner. It is nevertheless important to realise that very few human actions, if any at all, occur outside a political context, and that this context may be a predominant incentive to act in a determined fashion.

As a third element, it is useful to remember that power relationships occur in groups of various sizes, from the dyad of two people up to the complex interactions between nation-states or even between blocks of countries. Whatever the level of intervention in health promotion, be it the provision of individualised services in a neighbourhood health clinic or the design of health-related policies at the international level, it should be remembered that the political element is always present.

Finally, as should be obvious, politics, as used here, refers to power interactions which include, but go beyond, the mere horizons of party politics or electoral processes.

Health promotion. The definition of health promotion, proposed earlier, reflects well the current ambiguities of the concept as it stands now. On the one hand, in reaction to a field which has been very influenced by a behavioural orientation, it focuses too much on life-style modifications (Brown and Margo, 1978; McKinlay, 1975; Freudenberg, 1978, 1981; O'Neill, 1980; Labonte and Penfold, 1981; Watt and Breindel, 1981; Allison, 1982) the concept has significantly evolved in at least three areas (O'Neill, 1987a).

The first area of this evolution pertains to the legitimacy, in democratic societies at least, to use coercion in order to cajole people to adopt 'appropriate' behaviours. Whereas for decades it was assumed that people should voluntarily change their habits (Green *et al.*, 1980), it now appears more legitimate to use coercion, by legislative or other means, either to put on individuals the burden of their 'misbehaviour' (Knowles, 1977; Crawford, 1977) or to force corporations 'manufacturing illnesses' to produce less harmful commodities (McKinlay, 1975). This ethical issue in health promotion is by no means solved (see especially the whole issue of *Health Education Quarterly 14* (1), 1987), but it is clear that the legitimacy of coercion is more present than it was earlier. A second area of evolution pertains to who should educate whom. Whereas for many years it was perceived that professionals were the ones properly trained to educate the population, it has increasingly been admitted that a much larger range of people or organisations can become either the providers or the clients of health promotion endeavours. A third important evolution has also occurred: whereas the transmission of information was for a long time almost the only legitimate task for the health educator, it is now widely admitted that trying to influence the physical or socio-political environment into which individuals are evolving becomes a necessary part of the job.

On the other hand it can be argued that the conceptual evolution just described – which is also manifested in the semantic evolution from 'health education' to 'health promotion' that has occured since the beginning of the 1980s (in most Western countries at least), or in the push for a 'new public health movement' made by the European leadership in the field (see especially Kickbusch, 1986), creates a lot of confusion. Indeed, health promotion is slowly but surely completely absorbing the conceptual content of 'community health', another catch-all concept which emerged in the mid–1960s to take a certain distance from the older concepts of 'hygiene' or 'public health' (Conill and O'Neill, 1984).

As it has been argued elsewhere (Conill and O'Neill, 1984), that when a new rhetoric emerges like the current one about 'health promotion', it is interesting to understand: which interest groups promote it, for what reasons, and for whose benefit. Is it just a more or less conscious tactic of low-prestige community health professionals (trained in health or social sciences) to get access to social recognition and gratification (jobs, prestige, etc.)? Or, is it part of a larger social movement rooted in the economic conditions of increasingly huge segments of the population, proletarianised by the political economy of late twentieth-century capitalism? When one recognizes, in the changes proposed to health promotion, the leftist rhetoric of the 1970s emerging again in the midst of the 1980s – and promoted as well by conservative governments, as for instance the case in Canada (Epp, 1986a, 1986b), one has good reason to be a little cautious. Is not this renewal of interest for the social and political aspects of community health practice a kind of artificial niche created to promote a stimulating, but passéist, dream by progressive academics and professionals marginalised since the end of the 1970s but used by right-wing politicians for very different purposes?

Empirical evidence should be accumulated to document if this hypothesis about the political economy of health promotion evolution holds true. Is the 'new public health movement', orienting health promotion on more radical and more political paths, just a bunch of elegant words? Is it the most appropriate approach to deal with current health issues in advanced industrialised countries, especially in Europe? Depending on the answers to these questions, the meaning of the following discussions could be very different!

The lack of interest of most health promotion workers for the political dimensions of their job

In North America, at least, most community health practitioners show very little concern about the political dimension of their work. From what has been discussed for the USA (Freudenberg, 1981) and what has been analysed for the province of Quebec in Canada (O'Neill, 1987b), it can be argued that the reasons for this are ideological, technical and structural.

Reasons for this lack of interest. Ideological reasons refer to the quasi-moral reluctance of public health personnel, which in North America is mainly composed of nurses, to get politically involved. In general, as most people who work closely with them are able to realise, nurses enter their profession motivated by a type of 'service ideal' which is hardly compatible with the understanding of the world required to intervene politically. Being largely a women's profession which has its own peculiar perception of its role (Boston Nurses Group, 1978), politics is often seen by nurses as dirty and nasty; hence these professionals usually tend to negate the presence of social conflicts, given their 'do-gooder' orientation, and to leave to others the job of intervening in this area. These dilemmas do not concern nurses exclusively, most other professionals working in community health (physicians, social workers, etc.) are trained within the same kind of ideological framework.

Obviously, there are individual exceptions to this general situation. For instance, the extraordinary book of Nancy Milio (Milio, 1970), describing a slow evolution towards a more radical analysis and more political interventions, in her community health work in a Detroit slum during the 1960s, is a very good illustration of the moral and ideological discomforts a professional can go through when confronted by explosive situations.

Technical reasons. By technical reasons is meant here that, in their training, most health educators or other professionals doing health-promotion work do not learn the skills to analyse and utilise the political forces of their environment. It has been suggested that, in Quebec, the training received by community health personnel is biased towards epidemiology, biostatistics and medical care organisation, very little space being devoted in the curricula to the input of social sciences (O'Neill, 1987b). Analyses should be conducted in other provinces or countries, to see if similar biases are present; nevertheless graduate studies in the USA, as well as a long aquaintance with the international literature in health promotion, suggest that in North America it is the case, for at least two reasons.

First, the technical apparatus needed to develop the political skills of community health workers is not as readily available as the technical apparatuses of epidemiology or (bio)statistics. Indeed, the sciences producing the knowledge required to develop political skills (mostly social sciences like sociology, social-psychology, political sciences or anthropology) have reached less scientific consensus about what is an appropriate way of intervening effectively than other 'harder' sciences used in community health. Second, as many well known critics of the governmental service bureaucracies would argue (among others: Piven and Cloward, 1971; Leonard, 1973; Hasenfeld and English, 1974; Cloward and Piven, 1975; lllich, 1975; Helfgot, 1981; Lesemann, 1981), even if the capacity of these organisations to intervene more politically is often underestimated (O'Neill, 1986), their first and most essential function is one of social control more than one of radical, or even reformist, social change. It is not surprising, then, to realise that, in many countries, the skills and attitudes required to intervene politically in health promotion are not taught to the community health workers, who are clearly expected to help maintain the status quo rather than to challenge it.

Structural reasons. Finally, by structural reasons is meant that at the end of the 1980s, in a period of dismantlement of the welfare state in so many western countries, the service bureaucracies, in which much health promotion work is conducted, are fighting, not always successfully, to survive. Consequently the present time is not perceived by many workers as a good one in which to acquire skills which would make people and organisations even more vulnerable to critics and more exposed to cutbacks in scarcer than ever governmental monies; the author has realised that this is a widespread view, despite the fact that these very skills could help such organisations to devise better survival mechanisms for themselves.

A detailed case study, of attempts to develop more political health promotion interventions at the beginning of the eighties, has been conducted by the author on an important network of community health agencies in Quebec: the Community Health Departments (O'Neill,1986). Despite its idiosyncrasies and limits, this study empirically supports the statements made in the previous paragraphs, given that it also looked at similar processes in other networks of public services in Quebec as well as in the USA. We can thus admit that in North America, and probably in several other countries as well, the political skills of community health workers involved in health promotion policies or programmes are largely underdeveloped.

Political elements as hurdles for health promotion workers. This lack of concern is very sad, because the political dynamics of any milieu, which could be used to increase the effectiveness of programmes and policies, usually become a set of hurdles into which health promotion workers are likely to get trapped. In another paper, a series of four actual cases in health promotion, taken at various levels of intervention in the Canadian health system (local, regional, provincial and national), was presented to show how political factors like the marketing policies of a fast-food multinational chain or down-to-earth electoral constraints can counteract well-designed programmes or policies

(O'Neill, 1987b). In the same paper, another case was used to show, on the contrary, a clever utilisation of the political context which led a health unit to prompt a major change in a governmental policy, involving the treatment of thousands of acres of forest with chemicals potentially threatening to the health of populations.

Towards a different vision of health promotion. Given the mostly negative impact of political factors on health promotion work, it is necessary to modify our vision of what this work is. For most health professionals, it is still a kind of missionary undertaking, legitimised by a 'do-gooding' ideology and by state mandates, all this basking in an aura of scientism. It can certainly be argued, as the physicians of the early public health movements in Europe did, that community health work and its health promotion component are primarily political undertakings. Health educators or health planners, despite being a part of the very strong medical world, are social actors with very limited powers in an environment where people are imparted by several other actors, many of them much more powerful than community health workers. In fact, with little coercive capacities, these workers have to convince individuals or organisations to stop doing all kinds of things perceived as pleasant and constantly reinforced by the dominant culture (McKinlay, 1975); in exchange for these sacrifices are proposed vague probabilities, more often than not scientifically uncertain, of decreasing by a certain percentage the occurrence of a condition in the distant future. Seen in this light, it should not be surprising to observe that the lack of success of scores of health-promotion programmes is directly related to their promoters' lack of political power or political astuteness to promote them.

The vision of health promotion as a political process has often been confirmed to the author over the years through his constant interactions with community health personnel in Quebec (especially nurses); many of them, after analysing years of failures or partial successes of their programs (for their knowledge of epidemiology or programs planning), begin to find that this political vision is extremely useful to understand another way to interact, potentially more fruitfully, with their environment. Hence, it is mostly to design tools allowing these professionals and other people involved in health promotion to understand and use the political environment in their day-to-day work (at whatever the level they are involved within the system), that the project described in the following section was undertaken.

*Strategies to intervene politically in health promotion: the
ongoing story of an ambiguous research undertaking*

One objective, three assumptions. This ongoing project, on which
preliminary work was conducted from May to October 1986 has
one main objective: to develop a set of practical guidelines, presented in a book, to help people interested in health promotion
to analyse and utilise their political environment. To the author's
knowledge, despite a few exceptions among which Brownlea's
book (Brownlea, 1978) stands in a special category, there are very
few 'how to do it' books aimed at health promotion workers which
deal with political elements and their utilisation. In French, which
is the only language understood and used by most health promotion workers in Quebec, the situation is even more dramatic
despite the recent publication of an excellent 'how to do it' booklet
(Chapdeleine and Gosselin, 1986), which gives a fair place to
political elements but gives little explanation of *how* they can be
used. The need for such a tool is thus enormous.

This research undertaking is based on three assumptions. First,
it is an action-oriented rather than a classical academic endeavour
conducted for the sake of pure science. As shall be discussed later,
even if the author is tenured into a professional school and affili-
ated with an applied research centre dedicated to helping the daily
work of community health professionals, this assumption creates
all kinds of problems when one evolves in an academic setting like
a university.

Second, it is assumed that the presentation of political strategies to community health and health promotion workers should
be couched in the language and the framework of 'program planning' (Pineault and Daveluy,1986). Two reasons justify this
second assumption. On the one hand, the 'programmes' approach
to community health work has been strongly pushed in Quebec
since the reform of public health agencies in the early 1970s
(O'Neill,1982). It is the framework and jargon most workers
in the field are currently using and, in the author's viewpoint, is
a valuable tool to systematise interventions, as long as it remains
a tool to reach goals, and not an end in itself. Given the ideological reluctance of community health professionals towards political
endeavours, presenting political strategies in a familiar framework
with a familiar jargon is less likely to turn them off than existing
books of political tactics which, in addition, are more often targeted
to social workers than to health workers.

The third assumption made in relation to this project is that increasing the political skills of these workers is one of the areas where the disciplines of social sciences can contribute most to the evolution of health promotion practice. As a sociologist evolving for several years in the arena of community health, I feel that this undertaking has a strong potential usefulness as well as a kind of 'disciplinary legitimacy' in a world where physicians, nurses and natural sciences still define the universe.

Methodology. In order to prepare the book, and translate into usable guidelines the wealth of knowledge and experiences already available on this topic, a twofold methodology was devised.

On the one hand, a thorough literature review of the international literature has been planned in order to gather what is already known about political interventions in organisations and communities. We felt during the preliminary work conducted on the project that at least four areas of literature could be explored to generate theoretical as well as applied knowledge on the topic: (1) academic literature on strategic analysis and organisational behaviour; (2) academic literature on social movements; (3) academic and professional literature on community organisation; and 4) the militant literature of left-wing parties and unions, which often provide 'how to do it' books to their members in order to help them in organising various 'activities' (demonstrations, strikes, etc.).

The second way to gather information would be through in-depth interviews with a certain number of health promotion workers (be they in grass-roots or more formal organisations), well known in Quebec for their political skills and chosen by utilising the 'reputational' method to identify community leaders widely used by political scientists (Bonjean and Olson, 1964; Kadushin, 1968). These people would be requested to accomplish two sets of tasks: first, they would be asked to reconstruct the sequence of events, as well as their role in them, in one successful health promotion endeavour where they have been using mainly their political skills; second, they would also be requested to explain how they would act in front of a simulated case, and how they would solve it.

The objective of these two tasks is to gather sufficient theoretical, as well as experiential, material to devise a model for political intervention in community health and health promotion that could then be incorporated into the planning strategies currently used by people working in this field in Quebec.

Progress report: ongoing problems. The major ongoing problem with this project is its somewhat unusual status. Everyone to whom it has been presented, from government officials to militant people (on politically hot issues in health promotion), from professionals working in the field to colleagues in the university, agrees on the blatant need for the book this project aims at preparing.

However, funding for realising the bulk of the work up to now has been denied. The agencies funding applied research in the network of governmental community health agencies in Canada are currently experiencing cuts in their budgets; they have established priorities, which are generally geared towards a specific group (the elderly, for instance) or a specific problematic area (mental health, for example) and cannot provide money for a more general endeavour like the one proposed by the project. The agencies funding more academic types of work which have been approached see the relevance of the project, but find it too applied, not generating a sufficient amount of new knowledge and methodologically sound, but incomplete; they claim that once the model has been established, an experiment should be conducted to validate it before launching it in the hands of people. Given that these reactions from the funding agencies are legitimate, and that the strategy for financing the project will have to adjust to these realities, a few issues nevertheless remain.

First, although it can be admitted that an experiment would clearly help to improve the model as well as to test scientifically its effectiveness, one has the clear impression that many professional practices proposed to community health by the more institutionalised disciplines of epidemiology or management are not requested to provide the same type of evidence before receiving funding. Second, can we afford to wait yet another 5 years, (i.e. the time that such a design would likely require before the results become available for day-to-day use by the professionals), if we believe that the need is there and such a tool is expected? Finally, if it is not perceived that one of several legitimate roles for professional schools in universities is to spend some time transferring what is already known in science into usable tools for practice, who will perform this role?

Another order of problems related to this pertains to several ethical issues. Providing health promotion workers with political skills (if we assume for the sake of the argument that the strategies proposed in the project would effectively succeed in doing so) is in a certain way giving them a kind of 'weapon' that could be used in different, and not always unquestionable, ways. What if these new skills are used by professionals, they being (consciously or not) often the agents of social control, to manipulate the population even more into adopting lifestyles which are not necessarily wanted or necessarily more 'healthy', and if they diminish people's control over their life? What if these professionals, in a different way, use them to counter the effects of the dominant culture by manipulating people to adopt more radical and militant behaviours, not only against the dominant order but often against the population's own will? And, finally, what if they are used by various groups of the population to manipulate or attack the professionals and academics?

Conclusion

Despite the significant issues raised by this project, we have nevertheless the strong feeling that it should be pursued. As a result of the preliminary work conducted in 1986, a tentative framework on the utilisation of political factors in health promotion has been developed and published (O'Neill,1987b). Articulated on: (1) a strategy to analyse the political forces into an environment, and (2) a strategy to plan the political dimensions as precisely as the other dimensions of a programme (including the evaluation component), this framework is extremely simple and has not yet been validated. It was presented cautiously as such, but was nevertheless published because it is the author's deep conviction that something has to be done quickly to help health educators and others to integrate the political dimension in their work. This obviously does not eliminate the need for more thorough and more scientifically tested strategies; in the meantime, however, it will hopefully contribute to sensitise and better equip health promotion practitioners to deal with the political realities of their environment.

References

Alinski, S. (1969) *Reveille for radicals*, Vintage Books: New York.
Alinski, S. (1971) *Rules for radicals*, Vintage Books: New York.
Allison, K. (1982) L'education sanitaire: la responsabilite individuelle et la victime prise comme bouc emissaire, *Education sanitaire, 20* (3–4), 10–13.
Bonjean, J. and Olson, P. (1964) Community leadership, directions of research, *Administrative Science Quarterly 9*, 278–300.
Boston Nurses Group (1978) The false promise, professionalism in nursing, *Science for the People 3*, 20–4 and *4*, 23–33.
Brown, E. R. and Margo, G. E. (1978) Health education: can the reformers be reformed?, *International Journal of Health Services 8* (1), 3–25.

Brownlea, A. T. (1978) *Community, culture and care*, St-Louis: Mosby.

Chapdelaine, A. and Gosselin, P. (eds.) (1986) *La sante contagieuse, petit manuel pour rendre la sante communautaire* Montreal: Boreal Express.

Charter (1986) *Charte d'Ottawa pour la promotion de la sante*, OMS, Sante et bien-etre social Canada et Association canadienne de sante publique. Ottawa, Novembre.

Cloward, R. and Piven, F. F. (1975), *The politics of turmoil*, New York: Vintage Paperbacks.

Conill, E. and O'Neill, M. (1984) La notion de sante communautaire: elements de comparaison internationale, *Canadian Journal of Public Health 75* (2), 166–75.

Crawford, R. (1977) You are dangerous to your health; the ideology and politics of victim blaming, *International Journal of Health Services 7* (4), 663–80.

Epp, J. (1986a) *Strategies nationales en promotion de la sante*, Vancouver, Communication presentee a la 77e conference annuelle de l'Association canadienne de sante publique.

Epp, J. (1986b) *La sante pour tous, plan d'ensemble pour la promotion de la sante*, Ottawa: Sante et bien-etre social Canada.

Freudenberg, N. (1978) Shaping the future of health education: from behavior change to social change, *Health Education Monographs 694*, 372–7.

Freudenberg, N. (1981) The role of health education in changing the social environment: propositions for a public health strategy in the USA, *International Journal of Health Education 24* (3), 112– 19.

Green, L. W. *et al.* (1980) *Health education planning, a diagnostic approach*, Paolo Alto, Calif.: Mayfield Publishing Co.

Hasenfeld, Y. and English, R. A. (1974) Theoretical orientations to human service organizations, in Hasenfeld and English (eds.) *Human service organizations: a book of readings*, Ann Arbor: University of Michigan Press, 25–32.

Helfgot, J. (1981) *Professional reforming: mobilization for youth and the failure of social sciences*, Boston: D.C. Heath.

Illich, I. (1975), *Medical Nemesis*, London: Calder and Boyars Ltd.

Kadushin, C. (1968) Power influence and social circles: a new methodology for studying opinion makers, *American Sociological Review 33*, 685–99.

Kickbusch, I. (1986) Health promotion, a global perspective, *Canadian Journal of Public Health 77* (5), 321–7.

Knowles, J. H. (1977) The responsibility of the individual, *Deadalus 106* (1), 57–81.

Labonte, R. and Penfold, S. (1981) Analyse critique des perspectives canadiennes en promotion de la sante, *Education sanitaire 19* (3–4), 4–10.

Leonard, P. (1973) Professionalization, community action and the growth of social service bureaucracies, *The Sociological Review Monographs 20*, 103–19.

Lesemann, F. (1981) *Du pain et des services, la reforme de la sante et des services sociaux au Quebec*, Montreal: Editions Cooperatives Albert St-Martin.

McKinlay, J. B. (1975) A case for refocusing upstream; the political economy of illness, in *Applying behavioral science to cardiovascular risk*, proceedings of The American Heart Association Conference, Seattle, 7–17.

Milio, N. (1970) *9226 Kercheval, the storefront that did not burn*, Ann Arbor: University of Michigan Press.

O'Neill, M. (1980) A perspective on politics and health education policies, *Health Education 18* (4), 4–7.

O'Neill, M. (1982) L'intervention sociologique en milieu public et parapublic: application d'une problematique alternative au cas de la santé communautaire quebecoise, in A.C.S.A.L.F. (ed.) *L'intervention sociale*, Montreal: Editions coopératives Albert St-Martin.

O'Neill, M. (1986) *Innovative practices in governmentally funded community health agencies: the case of Quebec's D.S.C.'s*, Quebec; Centre de Recherche sur les services communautaires, Université Laval; 483 pages (No. 1 de la collection Edition Spéciale).

O'Neill, M. (1987a) *L'approche critique en promotion de la santé dans les Departements de santé communautaire quebecois*, Quebec; Centre de recherche sur les services communautaires, Université Laval. (No. 2 de la collection Rapport de Recherche).

O'Neill, M. (1987) Les contraintes imposées par les facteurs politiques aux interventions gouvernementales en promotion de la santé, *Hugie*, *4* (4), 32–7. Pineault, R. and Daveluy, C. (1986) *La planification de la santé, concepts, methodes, strategies*, Montreal: Agence d'arc.

Piven, F. F. and Cloward, R. (1971) *Regulating the poor; the functions of social welfare*, New York: Vintage Paperbacks.

Watt, A. and Breindel, C. (1981) Health education: structural vs behavioral perspectives, *Health Policy and Education 2*, 47–57.

World Health Organization (1986) Health promotion, a discussion on the concept and principles, *Health Promotion 1* (1), 73–7.

21

RONALD LABONTE

COMMUNITY HEALTH PROMOTION
STRATEGIES

Ten years ago, the big news in public health was 'lifestyles', an approach that sought to curb rising sick-care costs by targeting unhealthy individual behaviours for change. While this approach to health promotion has undeniably scored some successes and found a place in our popular culture, its limitations are also becoming increasingly evident. Poverty, under-employment and pollution are playing a growing role in the health problems of our society, and we are coming to recognise that neither lifestyles nor the modern epidemic of chronic disease can be viewed in isolation from our social, economic, industrial and political structures.

It is not surprising, then, that a 'new' health promotion rhetoric is emerging. The 1986 Ottawa Charter on Health Promotion (WHO) and Health Welfare Canada's discussion paper, *Achieving Health for All; A Framework for Health Promotion* (1986) challenge us to 'reduce health inequities' and to provide such health prerequisites as 'peace, shelter, food, income, a stable eco-system, sustainable resources, social justice and equity'.

While it is encouraging to see socio-environmental health issues assume such prominence, public health practitioners may be forgiven for asking, 'So what?'. It is nice to speak of empowering communities and building healthy public policies, but how is this new rhetoric to be translated into programme reality?

The remainder of this paper will attempt to answer this question by outlining a 'community health promotion planning model' developed during a 1986 Visiting Fellowship with the Lincoln Institute of Health Sciences in Melbourne, Australia. The model

235

is a fluid planning guideline identifying a number of strategies that 'bridge' the new health promotion theory with its practice. Many of these strategies are not new. Their effectiveness in a community health promotion programme will, however, depend on the extent to which they are mutually reinforcing.

Identifying problems

As health practitioners, the first challenge we face is this: exactly what is a health problem, and who gets to define it? During a workshop dealing with the community health planning model, participants were asked to name the three most important health problems facing their community. Their answers fell into three broad categories: medical, public health and socio-environmental. These three 'paradigms' can be characterised as follows:

Medical. Begins with the existence of a problem. Disease-based. Actions generally based on treating symptoms, eliminating illness and/or preventing condition from worsening.

Public health. Prevents the onset of a problem. Behaviour-based. Actions generally based on promoting healthy behaviours, starting early in the 'life-cycle' (for example, smoking-prevention programmes in elementary schools). Deals with 'well' people and tries to prevent them from becoming sick.

Socio-environmental. Attempts to create social and physical environments that nurture individual health and well-being. Social-change oriented ('healthy public policy'). The direction in which the 'new' health promotion is leading public-health practitioners. Actions are community-based, often involve political measures, and are not restricted to health professionals.

Not unexpectedly, medical and hospital-based professionals attending our workshop were inclined to see diseases as the major problem; public health practitioners gave prominence to health behaviours; and community workers believed that social conditions such as poverty and unemployment were the main problems.

In the community health promotion planning model, however, it is the communities that define their own problems and concerns. In fact, the first step towards 'empowerment' is to return to the community the power of definition. The staff of Toronto's Department of Public Health (DPH) worked for several years in a nutrition project with sole-support mothers in Toronto's Regent Park housing complex. The traditional public health approach to preventing malnutrition problems among welfare recipients would have been to develop an appropriate nutrition-education programme, presenting low-cost ideas for purchasing and preparing food. However, these women wanted a community garden, a 'hands-on' learning idea that gave rise to a range of novel food-related activities. The women had defined their problem, not as a lack of nutrition knowledge, but as a lack of control over food and living conditions generally. The DPH supported this definition and it was not long before the women themselves saw the need to develop their own education programmes on low-cost food purchasing and preparation.

A health agency's first response to a community-defined problem is usually to study its relationship to public health. This could mean carrying out a formal epidemiological study or supporting community groups in conducting their own 'barefoot epidimiology', a strategy that is popular among health educators in the United States (Frendenberg, 1984). But at what point can epidemiological evidence be judged sufficient to warrant public health action and involvement? This depends in part on the planning framework adopted. Currently, health practitioners and agencies subscribe to one of three planning models, each of which is grounded in a different 'ideology' or world outlook (Parston, 1980).

The predominant 'neutralist' framework assumes that power is equally distributed among different social sectors; the health agency's role is one of balancing between competing interest groups. The 'advocate' framework, implicit in the new health promotion philosophy, assumes that society is inherently egalitarian, but that some groups have acquired more power than others. Here, the agency's role to intervene on behalf of those who are less powerful. Although the 'activist' framework adopts a somewhat similar approach, it rests on the assumption that socio-economic structures are inherently non-egalitarian. Changing these structures, and not merely the conditions to which they give rise, becomes the longer-term goal.

Policy development

Policy is a consensus on the ideas that form the basis of action. It underlies decision-making at the international and national ('macro') levels, the provincial and municipal ('meso') levels, and at the individual health unit or agency ('micro') level. Most health practitioner involvement in policy development at the macro and meso levels will occur in the form of a health advocacy initiative. Micro-level policy development, however, is often a key step in the implementation of a community health promotion programme.

Policy should contain at least three types of statement. The first is a mission statement – a broad articulation of agency goals that precedes the actual development of the programme. Needless to say, mission statements are often easier to make than to keep. The DPH's mission statement, for example, is 'to make Toronto the healthiest city in North America'.

Policy should also include an action directive, a commitment of agency funds and/or staff. The DPH's 1984 policy report, *Housing and Health: Public Health Implications of the Crisis in Affordable Housing*, stated that departmental staff would participate in all 'interdepartmental committees and task forces dealing with housing policies'. The same report recommended that staff 'assist community groups who wish to take an active role in solving their housing problems'. This constitutes the third type of policy statement – the permission statement – which allows staff to work actively with community groups in developing broader-based approaches to socio-environmental health problems. Permission statements both empower and protect agency or department staff whose help may be sought by groups involved in community-defined endeavours.

Media promotion

The term 'media promotion' can refer to the production of materials such as pamphlets and posters, or to the organisation of health fairs, displays, special events, focus months, and all-out media campaigns and public relations efforts. Although somewhat akin to health education, media promotion does not usually involve group participation. Also, while health education increases a person's ability to analyse and understand a health issue, media promotion serves to raise general awareness levels.

In the new health promotion, community development is a key component of media promotion. When a Toronto community identified unemployment as a problem, the DPH canvassed groups working with the unemployed to determine what was needed. Based on the survey results, the DPH took on the task of raising awareness among physicians regarding the effects of unemployment on health, and encouraging them to refer unemployed patients to self-help groups, political action groups or counselling agencies. The mail-out sent by DPH to a sub-sample of Toronto general practitioners contained a pamphlet (prepared in co-operation with unemployment advocacy and counselling agencies) which emphasised the need to break the cycle of isolation and self-blame commonly found among unemployed people.

Physicians and concerned agencies evaluated the effectiveness of the project and, based on their comments, a longer pamphlet addressed directly to unemployed persons was added to the package. The second pamphlet deals with the economic and political factors creating unemployment (to minimise self-blame) and recommends political action as one means whereby an unemployed person can maintain a sense of control, and, by extension, remain physically and mentally healthy. DPH initiatives on the unemployment problem are intentionally modest, yet they fill service/information gaps identified by community groups. Co-operating with community groups allows health agencies to break large socio-environmental problems down into manageable sizes.

The sole-support mothers who organised the Regent Park Nutrition project used the media to help reduce the sense of self-blame typically felt by people who lack power. They had grown tired of 'macaroni and cheese' media stories portraying welfare families as hopeless and helpless. They were angered by periodic accounts of 'super-welfare' families who spent their waking hours scrounging for bargains, bruised produce and day-old bread, 'proving' that welfare benefits were adequate 'if people really tried'. Both images created negative stereotypes of welfare recipients: apathetic and incapable of change, or too lazy and coddled by 'government handouts' to make ends meet.

To provide a more positive picture of sole-support mothers, project organisers developed a sophisticated media strategy. Politicians and reporters from all media are now regularly invited to the openings and mid-harvests of the community garden, and guidelines for working with the media have been produced. Over the years, dozens of positive stories on the project have been filed. This example illustrates an often-overlooked approach to media promotion: generating new stories on health issues, rather than purchasing costly advertising space. For health practitioners, this might simply involve having the occasional lunch with local reporters.

Close working relationships with the press can provide enormous 'pay-offs'. A few years ago, the DPH's family-planning programme produced a coffee mug as a promotional gimmick to increase condom use among sexually active persons. The mug carried messages, such as 'Play it Safe', 'Use your condom sense', and 'Dressed for the occasion'. Although never officially released, the mug became front-page news for a week when the media caught wind of it, with such banner headlines as 'Condomnation!'. Across Canada and even in Europe, television, radio and newspapers picked up the story, providing more contraception publicity than the department could have purchased in a decade.

Health education

Health education can be divided into three broad streams: school, community and professional health education. Our concern here is with the latter two, and, more particularly, with an approach known as 'popular education'.

Popular education originated in the 1950s with the efforts of Brazilian educator, Paulo Freire, and his colleagues to teach the oppressed peasant population basic literacy skills (Freire, 1973). The learning often took place on the streets, in markets and on peasant farms. During the 1960s and 1979s Freire's approach came to be associated with mass movements for social justice and political change in Latin America. In Canada, interest in popular education began growing among international development workers during the 1970s, moving into the public health sphere around the time when the 'lifestyles' approach to health promotion came under critical review (Labonte and Penfold, 1981; Allison, 1981). Regarded as a life-long process, popular education emphasises active participation, breaks down 'teacher–student' polarity, avoids manipulation by experts, and emphasises the collective nature of learning. Most importantly, it stresses the need for social change as a means of achieving basic health.

The organisational outline of the OPHA-sponsored workshops illustrates the dynamics of popular education (Farlow, 1987). The workshops used a planning format known as a 'learning loom', in which the goals, objectives, activities and resources formed the horizontal axis, and participant experiences, analysis and action plans formed the vertical axis. The workshop goal was to increase health practitioners' abilities to work effectively on socio-environmental health issues, and it utilised a number of popular education techniques, including:

> *socio-drama:* after 'brainstorming' some of the role contradictions faced by health promoters, participants devised a short drama acting out their dilemma;
> *group drawing:* in which groups created large pictorial representations of the socio-health problems identified, as well as their possible solutions; and
> *sculpture:* in which a large number of participants assumed different roles within an issue they had analysed, illustrating

the respective power relationships in the form of a massive human sculpture. Popular education techniques also include photo-essays, slides, role-play, pantomine and song. Having originated among low-literate people, these approaches are less 'word-bound' than conventional adult education methods. However, their real value to health practitioners lies in the fact that they are fun and foster alternative ways of analysing complex social problems, regardless of the literacy level of the group involved.

In one exercise used during the workshop on the community health promotion planning model, participants were 'taken' on a guided tour during which they were asked to construct their ideal healthy community. Small groups merged their visions into collective drawings of such a community, and these served as focal points for discussion on health values. As a result, there was already a sense of group solidarity and some consensus on values before the workshop moved to a stage entailing rigorous political and economic analysis of health problems. This meant that when sharp disagreements began to arise over the relative importance of, for example, capitalist economics in creating poverty, participants could return to their idealised vision of a healthy community and the values they shared. Political differences thus became less a matter of self-concept (leading to strongly defended positions) and more a question of finding the best strategy to achieve group goals.

While popular education is only one approach to health education, its emphasis on strengthening communities and creating healthier social and physical environments makes it especially relevant to health promotion programmes that are aimed at 'empowering' communities.

Health advocacy

Broadly speaking, health advocacy can be considered in two ways: legislation that promotes health, and lobbying for healthy public policies. Most health advocacy is directed towards senior levels of government, and involve educating decision-makers about specific issues with the aim of obtaining political decisions that improve the health of the general public.

On the legislative side, the DPH has undertaken two health advocacy initiatives. The first will enact a 'right-to-know' by-law, giving workers and the public access to the names and known effects of potentially hazardous industrial substances being used in Toronto. There have been similar initiatives in the US, and at least one other Canadian city, Windsor, is implementing its own 'right-to-know' by-law. 'Right-to-know' legislation has long been advocated by workers and their unions, environmentalists and community organisations. All these groups, as well as representatives of business, took part in the lengthy consultation process that led to the development of Toronto's by-law. A second legislative initiative will significantly reduce work-place smoking in the City of Toronto, requiring all work-places to establish a smoking policy that gives the benefit of disagreement to non-smokers.

Political lobbying, the other form of health advocacy, is a strategy that is being adopted increasingly by health agencies and departments. It provides a means of showing the connection between lifestyle health problems, such as smoking behaviour, and socio-environmental factors, such as government tobacco policy.

The new health promotion charter and framework suggest the need for health practitioners to become active in a wider range of groups, including grass-roots activist organizations, social-welfare groups and coalitions. This helps to give community-defined problems a health focus while also broadening the base of institutional support for socio-environmental change.

Health advocacy means 'taking a stand' on an issue. In 1983, the Toronto Board of Health learned that a group of Nova Scotians was trying to prevent forestry-spraying of the herbicides 2,4-D and 2,4,5-T, which can be contaminated by dioxins. Members of the Toronto Board of Health had just toured toxic waste dumps on the Niagara River, at least one of which was leaking minute quantities of dioxins into Lake Ontario. Toronto had already banned the use of 2,4-D in city parks (except to control poison ivy) on the basis that potential health risks exceeded any alleged weed-control benefits. It seemed only logical that the Board of Health should play the role of a health advocate in the Nova Scotia herbicide case.

On two occasions, the Board of Health endorsed strong positions favouring the citizens and opposing Nova Scotia government policy. Up to that point, no government had spoken out on the issue; as a result, the media in the Maritimes gave the event wide coverage. Although controversial, Toronto's advocacy initiative gave the Nova Scotia group a strong moral boost. Board of Health and DPH staff also raised $10,000 to help offset court costs in the citizens' legal challenge against the forestry company, and used the opportunity to raise public awareness regarding environmental health. Perhaps the most important function of this form of health advocacy is that it legitimises the concerns and efforts of community groups that might otherwise be dismissed as 'fringe' by media or senior government officials.

Community development

Community development (CD) is the backbone of community health promotion. Two major modes of CD have emerged in the twentieth century. Although both have their roots in the Americas, they have influenced community organising internationally. One takes its inspiration from Chicago organiser, Saul Alinsky, while the other is based on the popular education theory of Paul Freire (Turner, 1985).

Alinsky defined 'community' largely in geographic terms and promoted 'them/us' confrontations in which 'they' were any persons not part of the organised group or living outside the geographic area. Emphasising the practical nature of single-issue organising, Alinsky was wary of forming coalitions with other groups. His technique entailed developing 'natural' leaders in churches, unions, and other community groups, forging a large, single issue 'organisation of organisations', and giving a 'face' to the community problem. 'Poverty', for example, might be embodied in a particular politician or business person who had resources and the power to actually change 'community' conditions.

For Freire, on the other hand, 'community' is defined more in terms of affinity of interest. His 'popular education' approach rests on a sophisticated analysis of oppression that takes into consideration broad sexual and class politics. It is an approach that supports coalition-building and favours the idea of working simultaneously on many issues. Moreover, it encourages the development of skills and powers of critical analysis among those involved in community-based organisations.

Each approach has strengths and weaknesses, and the current CD trend is to blend the best from both systems. Although Alinsky's confrontationist style of organising may be effective in many instances, it often places health practitioners in the uncomfortable position of mediating between those with power (for example, government departments) and those without.

A third, uniquely Canadian approach to community development uses film as a means of helping communities to organise themselves. In response to the recent influx into Toronto of Central American Refugees, the DPH produced a short film entitled *Salud* (Spanish for 'health'). The film showed newly-arrived refugees discussing health problems experienced in their native countries (often including torture), and since coming to Canada. *Salud* was used to bring members of the Spanish-speaking community together to explore the causes of their current Canadian problems and to work towards possible solutions.

In recent years, this same process has helped to create various community groups that have scored successes, such as the following:

> *developing* a full-service, bicultural, bilingual Multicultural Health Centre proposal, through an alliance of Portuguese, Czech, Korean, Salvadoran, Vietnamese, native Canadian and Russian communities;

> *participating* in the formation of a Multicultural Health Coalition, which has produced health information materials in twelve languages and sponsored conferences on multicultural health concerns; and

> *lobbying* the provincial government to lift restrictions on immigrant and refugee access to the health professions.

The DPH has eight community health officers and a number of education consultants and multicultural workers whose duties expressly include community development. However, most health practitioners have neither the time nor the specialised skills to work as a community organisers. Their primary community development role is to facilitate, rather than to initiate; they become resource persons for community groups developing themselves around a health issue or problem. This was essentially the role played by DPH staff in supporting the Regent Park Nutrition Project, which had as one of its goals 'to debunk the stereotype of sole-support mothers being unable to do anything constructive to help themselves'.

This project began in the summer of 1984. As part of its summer programme, The Regent Park and Area Sole Support Mothers Group (RPASSMG) and a graduate student in nutrition organised a series of community development activities related to food. These included the establishment of a community garden, trips to 'pick-your-own' vegetable farms, a feasibility study for a food co-operative, community participatory dinners, and a food-consumption and nutrition-knowledge survey, which revealed that lack of knowledge was not a major factor in the poor diets of sole-support mothers. Approached for project support, government departments, foundations, companies and private individuals donated food for the garden's 'gala' opening and mid-harvest celebrations, as well as garden soil, roto-tilling, mulch, seeds and plants. Also, a federal summer grant enabled seven people to be hired, three of whom were sole-support parents.

Each summer, three or four community dinners are held, attracting over 100 persons. These occasions are used to present ideas for preparing low-cost nutritious food, and to experiment with different types of meals (for example, vegetarian) and styles of ethnic cooking, reflecting the multicultural composition of the housing complex. The 'ethnic' dinners provide an opportunity to organise new immigrant women, and to defuse racial tensions in Regent Park.

This project, which represents a micro-level approach to macro-level problems such as poverty, unemployment and high food costs, has inspired three similar ones within Metro Toronto and another in Ottawa. To help other interested groups, project staff have produced a comprehensive organising manual that covers every topic, from developing the garden, preparing favourite ethnic recipes and choosing the best fruit and vegetable farms, to targeting politicians and foundations for money, arranging free bus services and conducting garden media events.

Community economic development

Most community development activities are geared towards improving equity in consumption. They assist marginal or less powerful groups to gain a larger share of those government resources that reach the public through social and welfare programmes. These programmes represent government's effort to redistribute income, wealth or other forms of social security after the fact, the 'fact' being the way in which income and wealth are generated in the first place.

Community Economic Development (CED) is a form of community development that increases community control over actual economic production. Its goal is to improve the quality of life of a community by developing enterprises that meet social and material needs, generate employment, create wealth that remains under community control, and foster self-reliance (Turner, 1985).

CED's roots can be traced to the British co-operative movement of the early nineteenth century, when social reformers sought viable alternatives to the extreme exploitation that was occurring as a result of industrialisation. Today, CED remains a 'third economic way', neither capitalist nor socialist, but blending the entrepreneurial strengths of the former with the collective responsibility and social accountability of the latter. Most CED enterprises involve some form of worker co-operative, and, although large-scale 'production' co-operatives are scarce in Canada, many function effectively in Europe and Britain.

There are more than 200 CED ventures in Canada, mostly located in rural communities. The largest and best known is New Dawn Enterprises, a community development corporation in Sydney, Nova Scotia, incorporated in 1976 as a non-profit umbrella agency to meet the economic, cultural and social needs of the residents of Cape Breton Island. Having begun with $30,000 in Health and Welfare start-up funding and $100,000 in private loans, New Dawn now has assets exceeding $12 million, controls $7 million in commercial and residential property, and operates several public housing complexes, including a 27-bed senior citizens' residence. It also runs two group homes and three dental clinics, and helps to fund new community enterprises (MacLeod, 1986).

A Community Employment Advisory Society created in Nanaimo, BC, in 1975, has since spawned a salmon hatchery, a squab farm, aviation and wood-working companies, a garden centre, and several day-care and optical centres. The borough of York, Ontario, established a CED corporation in 1978 which, between 1981 and 1984, increased its annual revenue from $2,000 to over $2 million. Its activities include the renovation of dilapidated buildings by school-leavers; the operation of a temporary employment business service that provides work for students in an adult day school; the establishment of ten parent-run day-care and nursery centres; and a multicultural theatre troupe and community opera (Shuttleworth, 1984).

Although these enterprises were created to enhance social rather than health objectives, their impact on health is obvious. They create jobs and thus reduce the effects of poverty and unemployment. They strengthen communities, often providing supportive social services that would otherwise not be available. In some instances, they offer affordable housing. Their co-operative approach reduces occupational stress levels and, by extension, the risk of occupational hazards. What is more, the fact of community accountability increases the potential of CED projects to be environmentally sound. In most CED ventures health practitioners are facilitative players. DPH staff have supported several initiatives in Toronto, providing assistance in funding applications and ideas for economically viable healthful enterprises, and liaising with other government departments.

CED is by no means a panacea, either for the nation's economic difficulties or for the poorer health experienced by socially less powerful groups. It does, however, offer a community approach to health promotion that begins to close the gap between economic production and social welfare consumption.

Government financial support is needed to create community economic development ventures that can become economically self-sufficient and increase community control over production.

Evaluation

Evaluating community health-promotion programmes is important for three reasons. First, the new concept of health promotion and its assorted 'frameworks' and 'charters' remain untested; second, because many of their concepts and methods are new, they still need to be refined by health practitioners, and evaluation will help to enhance the professional knowledge base; third, programme evaluation is often required as a condition of funding by governments, foundations and others who provide financial assistance to community health promotion programmes.

With health promotion moving into a socio-health paradigm, the selection of an appropriate evaluation design is critical. Clearly, community development efforts cannot be evaluated as if they were a new drug. Also, there is some danger that unrealistic expectations of CD programmes, buttressed by an inappropriate evaluation methodology, could actually 'prove' that a 'successful' programme had 'failed'. This applies equally to health advocacy initiatives, CED enterprises and, to a lesser extent, health education and media promotion endeavours.

At the community level, it can be useful to establish indicators of overall 'community health'. The Healthy Cities project is currently developing a number of such indicators. These include not only obvious ones such as socio-economic status and health status, but also various 'quality of life' or 'quality of community' measures, such as the amount of green space, crime levels, the availability of affordable housing, the level of political participation, and so forth. Data of these kind can reveal the health potential of a given socio-economic environment, as well as enabling us to measure improvements over time.

Social and economic factors can actually condition health behaviours and create independent health risks. However, there are also important psychosocial dynamics that should be integrated into the goals of community health promotion programmes. Improving social support networks, for example, can improve personal health (Berkman, 1984; Gottlieb, 1983). Decreasing self-blame and increasing people's perception of personal power and command of resources are also correlated with better health (Lerner, 1986; McQueen, 1986).

These new concepts are still undergoing refinement, but they promise to provide a rich source of information for health practitioners wishing to evaluate community health promotion programmes. Their significance lies in the fact that they begin to synthesise improved personal health and well-being with the process of creating healthier communities.

Conclusion

As public and community health practitioners move towards the ideal of 'Health for All by the Year 2000', public health concepts are continuing to expand. Already they embrace disciplines as diverse as political economy, philosophy, sociology, community organising and communications theory. This is at once exhilarating and frustrating. The range of potential initiatives is so limitless and the territory so large that almost anything is possible. Yet, a mandate to solve centuries of oppression and human foibles is in danger of becoming a mandate to do nothing.

The community health promotion planning model presented here offers a set of strategies that appear to work. It attempts to blend the constraints of community health practice with the idealism of the new health promotion. The model's essential message is this: health practitioners must become 'team players' in CD, advocacy, education, media and CED projects with other agencies, government sectors, and, most importantly, with local community organisations. Health promotion is no longer the exclusive domain or responsibility of health practitioners and health departments. The rules have changed; accordingly, health agencies must revise old policies and approaches.

By sharing our endeavours with an ever-widening network of groups, health practitioners can move closer to transforming 'Achieving Health for All' from an impossible ideal into a realistic goal. What is needed is commitment and co-operation in the task of creating healthy social, economic and physical environments and thus, healthy people.

Whether or not we label our actions towards this end 'health promotion' is largely irrelevant. The important thing to recognise is that empowering communities to take control of their health means giving them control over the programme. Community health promotion programmes belong, not to health agencies or departments, but to organised sectors of the community that seek support from health departments in their own endeavours to create a healthier, more equitable society.

References

Allison, K. (1981) Health education: self-responsibility vs blaming the victim, *Health Education 20*, 11–13.

Berkman, L. (1984) Assessing the physical effects of social networks and social support, in *Annual Reviews of Public Health 5*, 413–32, Palo Alto, Calif.: Annual Reviews Inc.

Farlow, D. (ed.) (1987) *Challenging our Assumptions: The Role of Popular Education in Promoting Health*, Toronto: Ontario Public Health Association.

Freire, P. (1973) *Education For Critical Consciousness*, New York: Seabury Press.

Freudenberg, N. (1984) *Not in Our Backyards: Community Action For Health in the Environment*, New York: Monthly Review Press.

Gottlieb, B. (1983) *Social Support Strategies: Guidelines For Mental Health Practice*, London: Sage Publications.

Health and Welfare Canada (1986) *Achieving Health For All: A Framework For Health Promotion*, Ottawa.

Labonte, R. and Penfold, S. (1981) Canadian perspectives on health promotion: a critique, *Health Education 19*, 4–9.

Lerner, M. (1986) *Surplus Powerlessness: The Psychodynamics of Everyday Life and the Psychology of Individual and Social Transformation*, Oakland Calif.: Institute for Labor and Mental Health.

MacLeod, G. (1986) *New Age Business: Community Corporations that Work*, Ottawa: Canadian Council on Social Development.

McQueen, D. (1986) Third Annual Report 1985–86. The University of Edinburgh Research Unit in Health and Behavioural Change, Edinburgh.

Parston, G. (1980) *Planners, Politics and Health Services*, London: Croom Helm.

Shuttleworth, D. (1984) Aiding the discarded generation: youth employment and community development, *Orbit Sixty-Nine 15*, 9–12.

Turner, S. (ed.) (1985) *Creating Community Employment*, Toronto: Ontario Community Development Association.

World Health Organisation (1986) *Ottawa Charter for Health Promotion*, International Conference on Health Promotion, Ottawa; Canadian Public Health Association.

22

ALF TROJAN

COMMUNITY ASSOCIATIONS IN HAMBURG AND THEIR SIGNIFICANCE FOR HEALTH

Introduction

The socio-epidemiological concepts 'social support' and 'social networks' have become core elements of the World Health Organisation's strategy for 'health promotion'. Starting from the recent developments in socio-epidemiological theory and health policies as well as from a former project on self-help groups (Trojan, 1986), we tried to assess the contribution of community organisations to health. This paper presents findings of a survey on 1,163 community organisations beyond market and the state, i.e. in the so-called 'Third Sector' or 'Non-Profit-Sector'. The first part describes two underlying concepts; the second part gives some information on the sample and methods of our survey; the third part presents the hypotheses of the study and some main results on health-relevant functions of community organisations in Hamburg. The final part of the paper deals with recommendations for action and demonstrates ways in which one could include community organisations into a 'healthy public policy'.

Social networks

Social networks are seen as an important resource for prevention (Caplan 1964). In socio-epidemiological research they are taken as the informal structure for coping with health hazards and stress. Badura (1981) distinguishes between personal, social and institutional resources. The focus of our interest is on 'social resources'. Other terms are secondary networks, community networks, small, non-professional or informal networks. Hamburg and Killilea (1979) use the notion 'informal social support systems'. This includes: families and relatives; neighbours; self-help-groups; and community organisations.

All these concepts have not been well defined so far; they overlap to a large degree.

Figure 22.1 gives an overview of informal and formal health promotion structures in the informal and formal sector.

Most studies on informal social support systems focus on 'personal networks', i.e. the focus lies on the individual as the centre of the network. We, however, did research on organised networks in the community. These community organisations are not centred around a person but rather around a task or common interest, therefore we call them task- (or interest-) oriented social networks. Single persons and their networks were not the object of our survey; they are, however, important targets of the activities of community organisations and will be discussed later. Another difference in our focus is that we look at the outward-oriented goals and effects of social networks, while most research (especially those of community psychologists) looks at the effects on the 'central' person, who is usually a person in need.

Social networks have functions which are relevant for health (cf. Trojan *et al*. 1987) These health-relevant functions can be summarised in the concepts 'social support', 'network promotion', 'empowerment' and 'social action'.

The Hamburg survey of community organisations

Our survey was to include all organisations in the 'informal sector', i.e. organisations which – first of all – are non-governmental and non-profit. By consulting a great variety of diverse directories, pamphlets, newspapers, etc. we found the addresses of about 1,700 organisations, associations and citizen initiatives. The large number of addresses itself was a remarkable result: it shows the quantitative importance of our research field.

Between May and August 1986 we sent written questionnaires to about 1,700 community organisations. A first part of the questionnaire enabled us to determine whether respondents fulfilled the selection criteria:

(1) non-governmental;
(2) non-profit;
(3) no restrictions for access;
(4) not primarily cure or therapy oriented; and
(5) not only temporary, but permanent, activities.

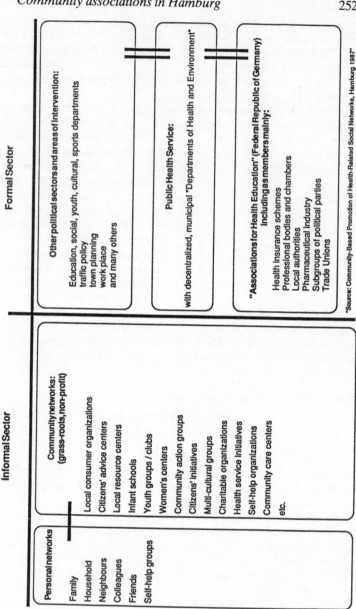

Formal Sector

Other political sectors and areas of intervention:

Education, social, youth, cultural, sports departments
traffic policy
town planning
work place
and many others

Public Health Service:

with decentralized, municipal "Departments of Health and Environment"

"Associations for Health Education" (Federal Republic of Germany)
Including as members mainly:

Health Insurance schemes
Professional bodies and chambers
Local authorities
Pharmaceutical Industry
Subgroups of political parties
Trade Unions

Source: Community-Based Promotion of Health-Related Social Networks, Hamburg 1987

Informal Sector

Community networks:
(grass-roots, non-profit)

Local consumer organizations
Citizens' advice centers
Local resource centers
Infant schools
Youth groups / clubs
Women's centers
Community action groups
Citizens' Initiatives
Multi-cultural groups
Charitable organizations
Health service Initiatives
Self-help organizations
Community care centers
etc.

Personal networks

Family
Household
Neighbours
Colleagues
Friends
Self-help groups

Figure 22.1. Health relevant structures in the formal and informal sector.

What has been surveyed?

Associations, community organizations and initiatives, which
- are non-governmental
- are non-profit
- have no restrictions for access
- are not primarily cure or therapy oriented
- are not only temporary activities.

population=1163 organizations and initiatives

The following organizations are included in the analysis:

    citizens advice centres
    counselling agencies
    leisure and hobby clubs
    community centres
    crêches
    citizen groups/initiatives
    charitable organizations
    youth organisations
    institutions for adult education
    cultural initiatives
    working groups
    peer groups
    multi-cultural groups
    immigrants'
    initiatives, community care centres
    and many more

473 (41%) organizations and
initiatives returned the
questionnaire.

Source: Community-Based Promotion of Health-Related Social Networks, Hamburg 1987

Figure 22.2. A survey of community organisations and citizen initiatives in Hamburg.

A number of areas, i.e. sports clubs, parishes, senior citizens, clubs were excluded, although they fulfilled our criteria. During the course of our survey we came to realise that these areas would have required special research instruments. Eventually we arrived at a number of 1,163 community organisations which were included in the survey. The diversity of these organisations is shown in Figure 22.2.

With respect to the response rate and representativeness of our survey, 473 (41 per cent) of the returned questionnaires could be included in the analysis. Responders and non-responders were compared with regard to two variables: postal code, i.e. the part of Hamburg they came from; and main activity area (information, which in most cases was recognisable from their names).

There were no significant differences in these two parameters, except that there was an over-representation of the 'psycho-social' and illness area, whereas the other areas were slightly under-represented.

From the evaluation of a large number of answers in the extensive questionnaire we discovered that most of the organisations pay attention to activities which directly or indirectly have a significance for health. We proceeded from two questions in order to differentiate between those with more and those with less involvement in health:

> 1. whether or not they have health matters as an aim for their activities, and
> 2. whether or not there is motivation for performing health related activities in the future.

In relation to the first of these questions, 65 per cent (309 organisations) declare that health is either a primary or secondary aim of their activities. These will be referred to as 'health-related'. About two-thirds of the health-related organisations would be interested in expanding their health promotion activities, provided that time and money were available. These groups will be referred to as 'highly motivated' health-related organisations. None-the-less, 23 per cent of the 309 health-related community organisations do not indicate that they would be prepared to expand their health-related activities. However, we can nevertheless suggest that these, too, may be relevant for health promotion. First, in the course of time, attitudes and work prospects of the organisations change and, second, it can be assumed that health would be more intensely pursued if sufficient incentives and assistance were offered.

From the 473 respondents, 35 per cent remain who declared health not to be an aim of their work. These are not considered any further in the following analysis. However, we wish to emphasise that by far the majority – i.e. the result of a corresponding question – consider their work as relevant for the health of their users and/or of society in general. Even half of the last 10 per cent of respondents, with neither health aims nor self-reported health effects, give some sort of social support. According to socio-epidemiological findings, this has to be considered important for neutralising and buffering stress; in other words, for the preservation of health. Henceforth, we will present the results only of the health-related community organisations (N = 309).

Areas of activity are numerous (Table 22.1). Organisations engaged in only one area are practically non-existent. Activities are recorded most frequently in the social area.

Table 22.1. Activity areas (n = 309)

(Multiple choice possible)	(%)
Social work	46
Psycho-social	42
Hobby/leisure time	30
Nutrition/good health	26
Education	25
Environment	25
Training/adult training	23
Community work	22
Disease	20
Addiction	18
Socio-cultural	18
Workplace	17
Peace	16
Human rights	15
Religion	12
Third world	11
Arts	11
Consumer rights, sciences, housing, etc.	23

Source: Community-Based Promotion of Health-Related
Social Networks, Hamburg 1987.

Table 22.2. Closeness to social movements
(n = 466). On average two indications per
community organisation were mentioned

	(%)
Self-help	24
Citizen	17
Health	16
Environment	15
Peace	14
Alternative	13
Women's lib	13
Youth	12
Human rights	11
Crêches	5
Labour	3

Source: Community-Based Promotion of
Health-Related Social Networks, Hamburg 1987.

Self concepts. It is not appropriate to summarise the organisations under 'self-help' groups since only every fifth regards itself to be a 'self-help group' or an 'association for mutual aid'. Help for others explicitly prevails over self-help. Also the question on belonging to a social movement revealed that a mere 26 per cent feel that they belong to the self-help movement. A total of 72 per cent sympathise with one or more social movements (Table 22.2).

By far the majority of organisations do not consider themselves to be part of the official care system (Table 22.3).

Target groups. An average of four to five target groups (Table 22.4) were reported. Of course, not all of the target groups can be reached equally well, but in most cases the target group can be contacted 'well' or 'very well' (40–60 per cent). Comparatively badly reached are immigrants, addicts, the handicapped, the chronically ill or other persons in need of care.

The large proportion aimed at the 'general public' can be explained from two angles. In the first place, it is contingent to turn to the general public on a large scale in order to reach the eventual user or supporter of the groups; in the second place, it indicates an unspecific approach, i.e. not selecting specific target groups or problems. Instead they have often a local orientation towards the 'general public' of a community.

Health-relevant functions of community organisations

Health goals. For a total of one-third of the health-related organisations, health is a 'central aim'. Almost all reported health effects of their activities for their users; almost three-quarters believe themselves to have a health-impact upon society in general. Some other health-related goals are: to educate for more health-conscious behaviour (40 per cent), to develop a 'holistic health conception' (37 per cent), and to convey a 'healthier perception of body and sensuality' (35 per cent).

Earlier we described our view that task-oriented social networks/community organisations are a 'hidden health promotion system'. This general concept was broken up into the following four research hypotheses:

    1. Community organisations are a source of social support for the community and for the target groups of their activities.

    2. Community organisations perform social actions in order to fight against health problems and health threats.

    3. Community organisations promote social networks.

    4. Community organisations are a means for empowerment.

In the following paragraphs we will examine to what degree our

Table 22.3. Closeness to official care system (n = 309)

	(%)
Part of the official care system	14
Complementary to the official care system	26
Alternative to the official care system	21
Nothing to do with the care system	39

Source: Community-Based Promotion of Health-Related
Social Networks, Hamburg 1987.

hypotheses were confirmed by the results of the survey.

Social support. The following items show how we operationalised the dimensions of social support (emotional, informational,
practical and material support; cf. Veiel, 1985):

    relief by conversation;

    contributing to the self-recognition of people who were
    'thrown off the track';

    offering sympathy, understanding, emotional support for
    people in need;

    helping with information or advice in cases of personal crisis,
    disease or other problems;

    informing about social conditions of diseases or health threats
    and how to face them;

    strengthening practical abilities;

    assisting other people in difficult tasks (such as the comple-
    tion of forms);

    helping people to receive financial or material benefits (such
    as clothing, accommodation, furnishing);

    helping people in trouble in other ways.

Almost all of the health-related associations reported at least
one out of the nine possible social support goals. Three-quarters
indicate that – according to their estimation – they attain at least
one goal 'well' or 'very well'.

Social action for better health. Health is a social category
which depends not only upon the necessary social support for
the individual but also on good living conditions: an environment
without pollution, a work-place without toxic substances, a society
which enables the development of self esteem and many other factors. Social actions aiming at the improvement of the environment
and life conditions in general have functions for the promotion of
health.

Work for a better environment, for example, extends beyond

Table 22.4. Target groups (n = 309)

(Multiple choice possible) (%)	Target groups	Main target group (%)
60	General public	38
49	Parents/couples/families	9
46	Youngsters	10
39	Elderly	6
39	Children	8
38	Immigrants	4
38	Handicapped	6
36	Women	6
28	Unemployed	2
28	Ill/in need of care	4
27	Addicts	5
25	Employed	1
22	Poor	1

Source: Community-Based Promotion of Health-Related Social
Networks, Hamburg 1987.

the organisations which have classified themselves as belonging to
the area of 'environment' (25 per cent). The second hypothesis
(social action) is confirmed to a lesser degree than the first, and
the following third, hypothesis.

Network promotion. Table 22.5 shows that community organisations want to support personal networks to a large extent. Items
of support for personal networks were:

> relief for or strengthening of families, partnerships;
> enabling friendships;
> organising mutual aid;
> increasing social contacts and communication in the com-
> munity.

But task-oriented networks are supported as well. It is most
interesting to note the immediate and apparent support which is
granted even to groups not belonging to the same organisation:
63 per cent indicate this in their answers. Most frequently, support
is offered in the form of advice, followed by letting rooms free of
charge. 78 per cent aim at founding and supporting new networks
or groups. In fact, new groups emerge less frequently: 65 per
cent of the organisations mention this. Thus, the organisations
contribute, to a substantial extent, to the preservation and further
development of this important sector of society.

Table 22.5. Working methods (n = 309)

	(%)
Individual consultation	83
Leisure time organisation	64
Practical help	60
Nursing/education	51
Care	17
Courses	60
Social group work	50
Study groups	43
Public relations	72
Protest actions	36
Lobby/committee work	34

Source: Community-Based Promotion of
Health-Related Social Networks, Hamburg 1987.

Empowerment. People seeing themselves and their lives as being dominated by the decisions of others and having learnt that their possible impact on their situation tends toward zero, are not very likely to increase control over, and to improve, their health. Referring to some aspects of 'locus of control' research, Rappaport (1981) proposes a strategy of empowerment for those in need (see also Berger and Neuhaus 1977). The intensification of empowerment, social activation and the experience of not being completely dependent on the mercy of others higher up in the hierarchy is decisive for good health. The neglect of this factor may be a reason for the failure of many of the health education programmes carried out hitherto, since they have not strengthened people but, on the contrary, have kept them dependent and thus made them even more helpless. Items for empowerment were:
  strengthening self-esteem;
  developing skills for self-help and standing up for one's rights;
  encouraging the collaboration of the afflicted for their common interests;
  mobilising citizen participation in politics and decision-making bodies.

Summary. Between 75 per cent and 85 per cent of all 'health-related' community organisations provide for social support, perform health-relevant social actions, promote other small networks and try to empower the population. These activities are identical with most of the subject areas which were defined in the 'Discussion paper on concepts and principles' of the WHO as the core of health-promotion. Community organisations (task-oriented networks) are a hidden health-promotion system. Promoting health means to a great extent strengthening community organisations.

Structural and organisational characteristics, co-operation, participation and demands for support of the community organisations will not be described within this paper. A summary of our results in this respect shows that they are: understaffed, underpaid, underfinanced, work under insecure conditions, use a large amount of time for co-operation and the gathering of information, and have a whole bunch of needs (e.g. support from local authorities, help with public relations, a voice in public bodies, organisational and personal counselling/supervision).

This leads to the conclusion that these social networks have on the one hand important empowering, supporting and health promoting functions, and on the other hand that they themselves need empowerment and support by public bodies. Health-promotion efforts, such as WHO's Healthy Cities Project, have to take into account the possibilities (and limits) of community groups, supportive and innovative potential for the better health of the community and its citizens.

Recommendations for policy

Healthy public climate of participation and responsibility. Our survey was on the one hand influenced by the changing focus of socio-epidemiological research from 'stress' to 'social support and social networks'. On the other hand our framework stems from the international discussions about health promotion and a new public health. These discussions were to a large degree generated and organised by the WHO. In the same month, when the first international conference on health promotion passed the so-called 'Ottawa Charter', we had a local conference in Hamburg – convening about 3,000 persons from community organisations and some formal institutions. The purpose of this local conference was to discuss the results of our study with the responding community organisations and other interested persons.

Our conference – under the heading 'Health is more' – confirmed what the main results of the survey were:

community organisations – regardless of their main activity area – are generally interested in action for health;

many of them would like to intensify their health-related activities and their co-operation with formal institutions;

most of them need support for their present tasks and the extension of health promotion activities.

One result of the conference was a heightened interest of the local health authorities in our research and in possibilities for strengthening health- promotion activities of the community. They ordered a consultative report on the significance of community organisations for health and some proposals for policy. The following suggestions are a summary of our recommendations to the health authorities in Hamburg (cf. Trojan *et al.*, 1987a). At the same time, we believe, these recommendations take up the ideas of the Ottawa-Charter. In many respects they are not only useful contributions but basic requirements for putting into practice what health-promotion action means.

Community organisations and their actions are an expression of a community's needs and problems, but also of its strengths and possibilities. Community organisations contribute – by the provision of support or through their pressure group activities – to all of the five areas of 'health-promotion action' mentioned in the Ottawa Charter. Community organisations are one of the most important actors for health promotion, so to say: a 'hidden health promotion system'.

Creating an infrastructure for strengthening health related community action: Local health promotion action and resource centres. As an intermediary structure between the big social institutions and city governments on the one hand and social networks and grass-roots organisations on the other, we suggest the establishment of independent local Health Promotion Action Centres, or Clearing Houses. Taking up the basic principles of health promotion (as mentioned in the Ottawa Charter) its functions should be:

enabling and initiating health-related activities of community organisations and other local initiatives;

mediating and networking between informal social networks at grass-roots level and health authorities or other formal institutions;

advocating for and supporting healthy public policy, e.g. organising campaigns – against toxic hazards, or for improving the quality of food.

This mediating body between the informal and the formal sector will have bridging and buffering functions (cf. Figure 22.3, middle column). The three functions correspond to the three basic principles of health promotion: enabling, mediating, advocating. The mediating body which is recommended here also represents

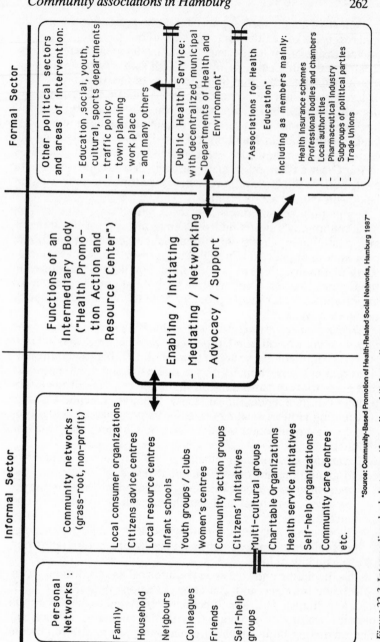

Figure 22.3. Intermediary body between 'formal' and 'informal' sector.

Formal Sector

Other political sectors
and areas of intervention:

- Education ,social, youth,
  cultural, sports departments
- traffic policy
- town planning
- work place
- and many others

Public Health Service:
with decentralized, municipal
"Departments of Health and
Environment"

"Associations for Health
Education"

Including as members mainly:

- Health Insurance schemes
- Professional bodies and chambers
- Local authorities
- Pharmaceutical Industry
- Subgroups of political parties
- Trade Unions

Functions of an
Intermediary Body
("Health Promo-
tion Action and
Resource Center")

- Enabling / Initiating
- Mediating / Networking
- Advocacy / Support

Informal Sector

Community networks :
(grass-root, non-profit)

Local consumer organizations
Citizens advice centres
Local resource centres
Infant schools
Youth groups / clubs
Women's centres
Community action groups
Citizens' Initiatives
Multi-cultural groups
Charitable Organizations
Health service initiatives
Self-help organizations
Community care centres
etc.

Personal
Networks :

Family
Household
Neigbours
Colleagues
Friends
Self-help
groups

"Source: Community-Based Promotion of Health-Related Social Networks, Hamburg 1987"

the necessary infrastructure for network promotion at the community level.

Some examples of health promotion activities that might result out of the work of such a kind of Health Promotion Action and Resource Centre, Clearing House, are:

neighbourhood forums and discussions on health-threatening living conditions in the area (e.g. toxic emissions, traffic hazards) and what to do to counteract and protect oneself,

initiatives working on improving the quality of meals being served for children in kindergartens/schools or for adults in factories and offices,

health fairs, bringing groups together and having an exchange of opinions and ideas,

neighbourhood play circles of parents and children,

working groups on specific topics and health problems, such as toxic hazards, AIDS, radioactive contamination, city planning, school situation, specific problems of ethnic minorities, and so on.

A local Action and Resource Centre for Health Promotion could meet the majority of needs and requests which were expressed in our survey (see Table 22.6).

Putting health on the agenda of community organisations: Health promotion contributing programme. To spread the idea of health promotion to a wider context and to reach grass-roots groups who are interested in carrying out specific health-promotion activities, a special programme could be helpful. Taking into account the Canadian experiences with such programmes, a fund should be created. Money could come from different sources (e.g. public funds, sickness funds, interested sectors of industry, social foundations, churches, and unemployment agencies).

The focus of the programme should enable non-profit community groups to conduct projects which they cannot finance themselves. This would increase public participation in health promotion and improve the capacity of these groups to develop health-promotion programmes according to the needs of their target population. As we found out, about half of all community organisations would like to develop more health-related activities if they had more money and other resources.

This programme could be an incentive for innovation and new ideas. Emphasis could be given to special topics or areas for a certain period, e.g. unemployment, toxic hazards, community development, nutrition, etc. (cf. Hildebrandt, 1987).

Table 22.6. Requests derived from the survey (n = 247)*

78% feel that new 'health knowledge' should be transferred from research and demonstration projects to independent institutions and initiatives.

74% think a forum necessary which fosters the exchange of experience and information on questions of health and social support.

70% asked for suggestions for health-related activities/health-promotive activities.

69% feel that more surveys are necessary on which health problems upset people or put them under pressure.

65% would like official institutions to co-operate more closely with community organisations and initiatives.

60% state that more organisational support is necessary for health-related activities or projects.

* Percentages refer to 247 community organisations which said, that they directly or indirectly are involved in health.

Source: Community-Based Promotion of Health-Related Social Networks, Hamburg 1987.

Opening health institutions for community participation: Changes within the health authorities. Although this is beyond the framework of our research, we would like to draw your attention to some necessary changes in the formal sector:

decentralisation of Health Authorities down to the district level (in Hamburg those institutions have just been renamed as 'Gesundheits- und Umweltämter', i.e. Departments for Health and Environment);

establishment of 'Health Advice Bureaux', meant to be the place where people with health problems can go, and as a starting point for health-related community work and long-term planning for a healthy community;

creating posts for 'Health Counsellors' or 'Prevention Advocates' in these bureaux for gathering information on local health problem and needs, and for passing the information on to the appropriate authorities and political institutions;

increasing community participation by giving more seats in local Health Councils or Committees to ordinary citizens, self-help groups, independent associations or other health-related grass-roots initiatives, thus improving direct democracy on a local level.

All these measures require that the public health sector takes

over a new orientation far beyond its traditional responsibility for
providing curative services, controlling vaccination or informing
on unhealthy behaviours. The responsibility for health promotion
has to be shared among many individuals, community groups, professionals, institutions and other actors. The public health service
can, nevertheless, have very important new roles: coordinator,
facilitator, catalyst, change-agent are but a few names for a new
self-concept of the future public health service.

References

Badura, B. (1981) Soziale Unterstützung und chronische Krankheit,
    Frankfurt: Suhrkamp.
Berger, P. L. and Neuhaus, R. I. (1977) *To empower people. The
    role of mediating structures in public policy*, Washington: American
    Enterprise Institute for Public Policy Research (AEI-Studies 139).
Blazer, D. G. (1982) Social support and mortality in an elderly com-
    munity population, *Am. J. Epidemiol. 115*, 684–94.
Caplan, G. (1964) *Principles of Preventive Psychiatry*, New York:
    Basic Books.
Deneke, C., Trojan, A., Faltis, M., Hildebrandt, H. (1987) Community
    organizations in Hamburg, BA thesis, University of Hamburg.
Hamburg, D. and Killilea, M. (1979) Relation of social support, stress,
    illness and use of health services, in *Healthy People. The Surgeon
    General's Report on Health Promotion and Disease Prevention*,
    Washington: DHEW (PHS) Publication No. 79–55071A.
Hildebrandt, H. (1987) *Lust am Leben. Gesundheitsförderung mit
    Jugendlichen. Ein Aktions- und Ideenbuch für die Jugendarbeit*, Frank-
    furt: Verlag Brandes & Apsel.
Rappaport, J. (1981) In praise of paradox: a social policy of empow-
    erment over prevention, *Am. J. Commun. Psychol. 9*, 1–25.
Trojan, A. (ed.) (1986) Wissen ist Macht – Eigenständig durch
    Selbsthilfe in Gruppen. In: fischer alternativ, Frankfurt/M).
Trojan, A., Hildebrandt, H., Faltis, M. and Deneke, C. (1987) Selbst-
    hilfe, netzwerkforschung und gesundheitsförderung. Grundlagen
    gemeindebezogener netzwerkförderung als präventionsstrategie, in
    Keupp, H., Röhrle, B. (eds.) Soziale Netzwerke, Frankfurt:
    Campus.
Trojan, A., Deneke, C., Faltis, M., Hildebrandt, H. (1987a) Gesund-
    heitsförderung im informellen Bereich. *Gutachten für die Gesund-
    heitsbehörde der Freien und Hansestadt Hamburg*, März.
Veiel, V. O. E. (1985) Dimensions of social support, *Soc. Psychiatry
    20*, 165–72.
Welin, L., Svärdsudd, K., Ander-Peciva, S., Tibblin, G., Tibblin, B.,

Larsson, B. and Wilhelmsen, L. (1985) Prospective study of social influences on mortality. The study of men born in 1913 and 1923, *Lancet i*, 915–18,

World Health Organisation (1987) *Health Promotion. Concept and Principles in Action: A Policy Framework*, Copenhagen: WHO.

World Health Organisation (1986) *Ottawa Charter for Health Promotion*, Ottawa: WHO.

23

JEAN SPRAY AND KAREN GREENWOOD

THE PROGRESS OF A COMMUNITY DEVELOP-
MENT APPROACH IN ONE HEALTH DISTRICT:
FROM STREET WORK TO DISTRICT POLICY

The Health Promotion Department of Paddington and North Kensington Health Authority appointed a Community Development Health Education Officer (CDHEO) in 1980. This was a new and untried post, which was created as a response to current thinking in health education, that health education practice needed to respond to the growing evidence that there were social and environmental causes of ill health, as well as those caused as a result of individual behaviour.

The CDHEO had a background of health visiting in the local area, and had already been involved in two successful local community projects whilst health visiting: Paddington Girls Project and a Women's Health Course at a local community centre. These two projects had brought her into contact with many local youth and community workers and she built on these contacts and influenced the subsequent development of the work, mainly with women's groups and youth groups, both mixed and single sex.

Over three years there was a sustained development of work and a gradual process of networking in the area, almost always working through other community and youth workers both in the voluntary and statutory sectors. Most of these workers saw the need for a trained health worker to contribute to these projects; many expressed anxiety, not only about their own lack of knowledge in the area of health issues and services but equally how they had been wary of asking for help from the Health Service, because of what they felt were inappropriate attitudes and approaches of health professionals towards the groups that they were involved with. The

CDHEO offered an opportunity for accessability, a willingness to adapt to local situations and the security of a sound knowledge base in health.

The work fell into three main styles:

1. *Work in community centres*, which involved working with several different groups who used the centres, for example, mother and toddler, coffee-drop-in group. These were often well-established groups that the community worker had been working with over a long period of time and who wanted a one-off session on, say, contraception or cervical and breast cancer, or wanted to plan several sessions with the Health Education Officers (HEOs) on children's health.

2. *Work with groups*, which is established by community workers outwith community centres. Again, this could involve one-off sessions or a planned programme/project over several weeks.

3. *Work with local residents and community workers* to establish a major local event around health in response to developmental work in an area, examples of these were women's health courses, alternative health therapies, 'Know your Health Service' courses.

The work of the HEOs began to have an effect on the Health Education Department after the first 4–6 months when the work became established and consequently experiences and needs were fed back to the department. These particularly influenced the training programme and the resources in the department.

The HEO resources officer (training) and the CDHEO began to work closely together. It became apparent that resource materials in the department for use with young people, particularly around aspects of sexuality and contraception, and resources on aspects of women's health, were thin on the ground; those that did exist were often out-of-date and not relevant to the setting of small-group community-based work. This led to a review of these resources which were held in the department and the production of a Women's Health catalogue in 1984.

The training HEO began to re-orientate programmes that were being offered to professional health workers within the district. Examples of this are: setting up of workshops which brought together health workers with community organisations, who were also providing services such as mental health organisations; providing training for health workers with the Child Poverty Action Group on welfare health rights and low-income families.

Through the work of the CDHEO, the department began to be

used more as it became known as an accessible resource, particularly for video and television hire and the use of graphics material and the library.

Some health visitors began to show an interest in the prospect of more organised, varied and supported group work. The department negotiated with the then Director of Community Nursing jointly to support an 18-month action research project by a health visitor who would work exclusively with community groups.

The research examined community work methods and health visiting and was produced as *Working in a Different Way* in 1985. This research has proved to be important and original work in the health-visiting field; many projects and practice methods have since been based on the work. It was significant that the work was done from a Health Education Department base; the advantages and lessons to be learned from this are documented in the report. The success of the project also influenced the manager of Primary Care Services to create a permanent post for a health visitor working with community groups who is also based with the Health Promotion Department.

This health visitor is of Afro-Caribbean origin and has chosen to work with black and other ethnic groups as a priority. Consequently, the department is benefiting from the development of new resources and more departmental contact work from different groups in the community.

The department also provides a base for the Community Dietitian who is similarly both benefiting from being located in the department and is benefiting the department through the development of resources, strengthening and widening community contact for the department and contributing to the development of the district food policy, which is co-ordinated from within the Health Promotion Department.

We are now at the stage of policy development with regard to our Community Development activities when we believe we must look at the growing number of health professionals within the district who carry, within their job description, some responsibility to do community orientated work, and offer a health promotion support and development programme to those individuals.

Currently this would include:
  A Health Visitor working with black and ethnic minority groups;
  A Community Dietitian;
  A Community Pharmacist;

A Parentcraft Co-ordinator;

Two Health Visitors working with a Cumberledge (neighbourhood nursing) project; and

Two Health Workers working with a care team for homeless families

There is also potential for those people employed within the district who are currently seconded to study for the Certificate in Health Education, which is designed to enhance health promotion within their professional work, to join such a programme. However, all graduates from this course do not have opportunity for community group work activity.

The development and support programme will initially be called a Community Forum and will set out to enhance the following skill areas:

Group work

Teaching

Presentation

Management of work

Writing

Evaluation

Understanding the Community Profile

In this section we describe the steps which the department has taken over the last year (1987) to incorporate the work described above into the policy-planning process in the district.

The work of the Health Promotion Department has taken place in a context of significant policy developments in the country:

1. In the early 1980s several health authorities began to develop health promotion policies which were aimed at the National Health Service (NHS) itself, but which also aimed to influence other public sectors (education, local authorities) and the community in general. Examples of these policies are: Food for Health, No-Smoking, Alcohol at Work, Exercise.

2. The WHO Strategy for Europe, Health for All in the Year 2000', was launched in the mid–1980s. This strategy emphasised the need to reduce inequalities, involve the community in its health care, and co-ordinate health promotion across statutory and voluntary sectors. An aim of this strategy is the reorientation of health services towards an emphasis on public health promotion. The UK is a signatory to the WHO Strategy, and Paddington and North Kensington District has also voiced its support.

3. Both the above developments have taken place at a time

of increasing interest in public health. In July 1987 the Public Health Alliance was formed to bring together people who are involved in public health.

The Health Promotion Department recognised the need to consolidate and take forward the work of providing professional support and training for field-workers to enable them to work in a community-sensitised way. This method of working is being incorporated into the strategy for Health Promotion for the Paddington and North Kensington District.

In July 1987 the first meeting was held of a new group formed to provide planning advice to the Head of Health Promotion Department. The intention was to have a group which had representation from the NHS (including operational managers), local authorities and the voluntary sector. The progress towards achieving such a grouping has been slow. The problems associated with forming the group reflect the difficulties of co-ordinating work within and across sectors.

Fieldworker input. NHS representation on the group is from Health Promotion, Community Medicine and Unit Management. The issue of how fieldworkers feed their voice into the policy-making process still needs to be addressed.

Voluntary sector involvement. The history of community participation in the NHS has largely been confrontational and, with a few exceptions, tokenistic. Particular problems arise when the voluntary sector try to place accountable representatives on groups in the NHS, which does not have an understanding of local accountability. The only formal mechanism for making the community's voice heard has been through the Community Health Councils (CHCs), which have limited resources and are widely recognised as having limited powers.

District Health Authorities are usually remote bodies with the consequence that many groups in the community have very little understanding of the NHS, how it works and how to make their voice heard. We have invited representation on the group from the CHC and the two umbrella voluntary organisations (councils of voluntary service). It is clear that for this representation to be more than tokenistic it is also important to take time to explain the nature of the group, the scope of its work and how it fits into the district structure.

Local authority representation. The district covers part of two local authorities: Westminster, and Kensington and Chelsea. There has been very little joint work between the Health Promotion Department (HPD) and the local authorities.

The mechanism for collaboration between the District Health Authority and the Local Authority is through the cumbersome structure of the Joint Consultative Committee. In terms of representation on the group it has been difficult to identify who to invite in the absence of health liaison units in either authority. Consultation over the strategy for health promotion may provide a means of developing collaboration and determining opportunities for joint work.

The first task of the group has been to advise the HPD on producing a strategy for health promotion. The strategy is based on the aims of 'Health for All'. The principles underlying the strategy are: reducing inequalities in health; being sensitive to community needs by explaining what those needs are; fostering collaboration between the NHS and other statutory and voluntary agencies to develop a comprehensive health promotion strategy. This was completed in March 1988. The document focuses on core activities of health promotion: professional support and development of fieldworkers; implementing district health promotion policies; campaign work/public education; training; resources.

Objectives for the department will be developed through consultation with care teams/planning groups in the NHS, local authorities, education and the voluntary sector and would be based on the core activities above.

There is no doubt that in inner-city and urban areas there is a trend for community-health professionals, employed by local health authorities, to be given posts whose job descriptions involve 'working in a different way' within their professional activity, in the hope that this will produce more community-sensitive and sensitised work practice.

This trend within health authorities has run alongside the development, over the last 10 years, of community health projects and the employment of community health workers outwith the NHS. The history and detail of this can be traced through the work of the London Community Health Resource and the Community Health Initiatives Resource Unit, who amalgamated in September 1987 to become The National Community Health Resource.

The growth of this new community development or community-sensitive work within the NHS has been piecemeal, appearing often as isolated individuals employed to work in a different way, either as a response to crisis in service delivery or as small groups employed on innovative projects which may be action-researched based and time-limited.

All of this change, in practice, is taking place in the wider policy environment of changes towards community care/consumerism – the promotion of self-help, locality planning, encouraging closer links with the voluntary sector, which is evident within the NHS at the present. In addition, there are notions being promoted of 'healthy cities' and 'health for all by the year 2000'.

What we hope to do from our small base, and with some experience of practice and process, is to take account of those changes and developments and provide a support for those individuals, within our sphere of influence, to enable them to feel confident in their roles and to liberate their skills and experience to work more effectively for and in the community.

References

Drennan, V. (1985) *Working in a Different Way*.
Drennan, V. (1986) *Effective Health Education in the Inner City*.
  Both are available from: Paddington and North Kensington Health Promotion Department, 287 Harrow Road, London W9 3RL.

Community Health Initiatives

24

JOHN ASHTON

CREATING HEALTHY CITIES

Introduction

In 1984 a conference entitled 'Beyond Health Care' was held in Toronto at which the idea of Healthy Cities was first put forward. The conference marked the 10th anniversary of a report by the Canadian Minister of Health, Marc Lalonde, entitled *A New Perspective on the Health of Canadians*. This report focused attention on the scope for the prevention of ill health in Canada. It is arguable that it signalled the turning point in efforts to rediscover public health in developed countries (Lalonde, 1974).

Since 1974, many countries have published similar prevention-orientated documents, the World Health Organisation has developed its strategy of 'Health For All By the Year 2000', there has been an explosion of interest in preventive medicine and health promotion and people have begun to talk seriously about the new public health movement (WHO/EURO, 1981; WHO Geneva, 1981). The Healthy Cities project is a major initiative to support the development of that new movement. The project is based on a recognition of the importance of the city as a living place for humans and as a setting which can have a profound influence on the achievement and maintenance of good health.

'Health For All By the Year 2000'

In 1981 the World Health Assembly adopted a global strategy of 'Health For All by the year 2000' (HFA 2000). According

276

to this strategy the aim is that in 15 years time all people in all countries should have at least such a level of health that they are capable of working productively and of participating actively in the social life of the comunity in which they live. The three main objectives of the strategy are to promote healthy lifestyles, to prevent preventable conditions and to enable the rehabilitation of those whose health has been damaged. Within Europe this strategy has led to the thirty-three member countries agreeing a set of targets as steps on the path to 'Health For All' (Table 24.1) (WHO, 1986a).

The European programme is intended to achieve a shift away from a narrow medical view of health towards an understanding of the social aspects of health through an expansion in five areas:

1. Self-care.

2. Integration of medical care with other related activities such as education, recreation, environmental improvements and social welfare (so-called intersectoral action).

3. Integrating the promotion of good health with preventive medicine, treatment and rehabilitation.

4. Meeting the needs of under-served groups.

5. Community participation.

Health promotion – a new concept for the new public health

Out of the arguments and discussions generated by the World Health Organisation Strategy a new concept has emerged; the concept of 'health promotion' (WHO Copenhagen, 1984). It is clear from our understanding of the way in which health improved in the past that if we are to achieve the potential for good health which is possible, a broad-based approach will be necessary. From this perspective health promotion as the means to 'Health for All' is seen as a process of enabling people to increase control over and improve their health. Health itself is seen as a resource for everyday life rather than an end in itself (Kickbusch, 1986).

Principles of health promotion. The experience of those active in this field since 1974 has helped to define five principles of health promotion.

(i) It actively involves the population in the setting of everyday life rather than focusing on people who are at risk for specific conditions and in contact with medical services.

(ii) It is directed towards action on the causes of ill health.

(iii) It uses many different approaches which combine to improve health. These include education and information,

Table 24.1. Targets For Health For All By The Year 2000.

Targets 1–12 – Health For All.
1. Equity in health.
2. Adding life to years.
3. Better opportunities for the disabled.
4. Reducing disease and disability.
5. Eliminating measles, polio, neonatal tetanus, congenital rubella, diptheria, congenital syphilis and indiginous malaria.
6. Increased life expectation at birth.
7. Reduced infant mortality.
8. Reduced maternal mortality.
9. Combating diseases of the circulation.
10. Combating cancer.
11. Reducing accidents.
12. Stopping the increase in suicide.

Targets 13–17 – Lifestyles Conducive to Health For All
13. Developing Healthy Public Policies.
14. Developing social support systems.
15. Improving knowledge and motivation for healthy behaviour.
16. Promoting positive health behaviour.
17. Descreasing health-damaging behaviour.

Targets 18–25 – Producing Healthy Environments
18. Policies for healthy environments.
19. Monitoring, assessment and control of environmental risks.
20. Controlling water pollution.
21. Protecting against air pollution.
22. Improving food safety.
23. Protecting against hazardous wastes.
24. Improving housing conditions.
25. Protecting against work-related health risks.

Targets 26–31 – Providing Appropriate Care
26. A health care system based on primary health care.
27. Distribution of resources according to need.
28. Re-orientating primary medical care.
29. Developing teamwork.
30. Co-ordinating services.
31. Ensuring quality of services.

Targets 32–38 – Support for Health Development
32. Developing a research base for Health For All.
33. Implementing policies for Health For All.
34. Management and delivery of resources.
35. Health information systems.
36. Training and deployment of staff.
37. Education of people in the non-health sector.
38. Assessment of health technologies.

---

community development and organisation, health advocacy and legislation.

(iv) It depends particularly on public participation.

(v) Health professionals – especially those in primary health care – have an important part to play in nurturing health promotion and enabling it to take place.

At the 1986 Ottawa Conference on Health Promotion these principles were taken further and developed as the Ottawa Charter for Health Promotion (WHO 1986b). The Charter stresses in particular the necessity to:

Build public policies which support health: Health promotion goes beyond health care and makes health an agenda item for policy makers in all areas of governmental and organisational action. Health promotion requires that the obstacles to the adoption of health promoting policies be identified in non-medical sectors together with ways of removing them. The aim must be to make the healthier choices the easier choices

Create supportive environments: Health promotion recognises that both at the global level and at the local level human health is bound up with the way in which we treat nature and the environment. Societies which exploit their environments without attention to ecology, reap the effects of that exploitation in ill health and social problems. Health cannot be separated from other goals and changing patterns of life, work and leisure have a definite impact on health. Health promotion therefore must create living and working conditions that are safe, stimulating, satisfying and enjoyable.

Strengthen community action: Health promotion works through effective community action. At the heart of this process is communities having their own power and having control of their own initiatives and activities. This means that professionals must learn new ways of working with individuals and communities – working for and with rather than on them.

Develop personal skills: Health promotion supports personal and social development through providing information, education for health and helping people to develop the skills which they need to make healthy choices. By doing so it enables people to exercise more control over their own health and over their environments. Making it possible for people to learn throughout life, to prepare themselves for all of its stages and to cope with chronic illness and injuries is essential. This has to be assisted in school, home, work and in community settings.

Reorientate health services: The responsibility for health promotion in health services is shared among individuals, community groups, health professionals, medical care, bureaucracies and governments. They must work together towards a health care system which contributes to the pursuit of health.

The role of the medical sector must develop towards health promotion beyond its responsibility for providing treatment services. To do this it will need to recognise that most of the causes of ill health lie outside the direct influence of the medical sector and be willing to work with those in a position to influence these causes.

From a historical point of view it seems that we have just entered a new phase in our way of thinking about health. The Public Health Movement of the last century was in time eclipsed by a more individualistic medical approach. As the most pressing environmental problems were brought under control, action to improve the health of the population moved on first to personal preventive medical services such as immunisation and family planning and later to therapeutics spurred on by the advent of antibiotics. It has been the impact of the McKeown analysis together with growing disillusionment at the escalating costs and diminishing returns associated with the treatment era which has in part been responsible for the renewed interest in preventive medicine and health promotion. It has begun to seem possible to plan for health rather than just planning to treat disease.

The new public health

What is emerging as the new public health is an approach which brings together environmental change and personal preventive measures with appropriate therapeutic interventions especially for the elderly and disabled. However, the new public health goes beyond an understanding of human biology and recognises the importance of those social aspects of health problems which are caused by lifestyle. In this way it avoids the trap of blaming the victim. Many contemporary health problems are therefore seen as being social rather than solely individual problems; underlying them are concrete issues of local and national public policy which local government in particular is in a strong position to change or influence.

In establishing the Healthy Cities Project as a major new initiative, WHO believes that the cities now, as in the past, have been the potential for effective pioneering action and that the time is right to support processes which are already in evidence in many European cities.

The healthy cities project. The Healthy Cities project is intended to lend support to city-based health promotion. The project is a collaborative one between the Health Promotion and Environmental Health sections of the European office of WHO. In establishing the project the experience of 5 years of health promotion development in the Mersey Region has been heavily drawn upon. (Ashton *et al*. 1986a). By bringing together a network of European towns and cities to collaborate in the development of new health promotion initiatives, not only will the cities learn from each other but they will play an important part in the dissemination of ideas and the establishment of the 'new public health'. By concentrating on concrete examples of health promotion based on community participation and intersectoral action, the Healthy Cities Project is seen as marking the point at which the 'Health For All Strategy' is taken off the shelves and into the streets of European cities.

The healthy city. Defining the healthy city is not an easy task; certainly a healthy city is more than one which has good health services. The concept implies that the city as a place which shapes human possibility and experience has a crucial role to play in determining the health of those living in it. Yet each city is unique and has a life of its own, a soul, a spirit, even a personality. To understand a city it has to be both understood as a complete entity and experienced as a place for living. According to Hancock and Duhl (1986) 'a healthy city is one that is continually creating and improving those physical and social environments and expanding those community resources which enable people to support each other in performing all the functions of life and in developing themselves to their maximum potential'. Central to such a definition is the social implication that in a healthy city there is some kind of agreed 'common gameboard' and that, broadly speaking, the citizens are pulling in a similar direction; however conflict and its creative resolution are also part of a healthy city (Hancock and Duhl, 1986). At its most fundamental, a city is unhealthy if it cannot provide its citizens with the basic resources for health: safe and adequate food; a safe water supply; sanitation; shelter; freedom from poverty. However, it is clear that these alone are insufficient and that a range of environmental prerequisites (economic, physical, social and cultural) are incorporated into what most people expect for themselves and their families if they are to enjoy full health in the city.

For most of recorded history, cities have actually been very unhealthy places in which to live, especially for their poorer citizens. It was as a result of the recognition of the relationship between poor housing and physical environments and the high mortality rates in the industrial cities that the public health movement of the last century came into being. It is no coincidence that urban planning had its origins in public health; nor that in some countries there often are or have been very close links between national ministries of health, housing, environment and culture.

The sheer awfulness of much of city life in the last century inspired many thinkers to consider what a Utopian city might consist of. To Ward-Richardson in 1875 such a city would have included clean air, public transport, small local hospitals, community homes for the elderly and mentally ill, no tobacco or alcohol and the adoption of occupational health measures. His ideas influenced the town planner Ebenezer Howard who developed the first 'garden city' suburbs in Britain in the 1890s as a technical solution to the slum city areas. Undoubtedly the influence of Howard at that time was an important one. However, it seems that the failure to consider technical solutions to human problems from the point of view of those directly affected has contributed to the large-scale planning disasters in the post-war period in many European countries. In creating a new public health, the paternalism which runs through much of this recent history, has no part to play.

The parameters by which one might measure the health of a city clearly span from the traditional ones of environmental protection and the quality of the physical environment through measures of mortality, morbidity, the quality of treatment and preventive medical services into much softer, though no less important, measurements which define culture, participation, intersectoral collaboration and levels of mutual support (Vertio 1986). A preliminary list of indicators of a healthy city might include the following:

Demography.

Quality of the physical environment including pollution, quality of the infrastructure and housing.

State of the local economy including unemployment levels.

Quality of the social environment including levels of psycho-social stress and quality of social support services, strength and nature of the local culture.

Personal safety.

Aesthetics of the environment and the quality of life.

Appropriate education.

Extent of community power and participation, structures of government.

Extent of intersectoral collaboration and emphasis on healthy public policy.

New Health Promotion Indicators, e.g. participation in physical exercise, dietary habits, alcohol and tobacco use.

Quality of health services.

Traditional Health Indicators (mortality and morbidity).

Equity.

The description of the health of a city along these lines requires a multi-disciplinary approach and a recognition of the validity of subjective data.

Healthy cities and the new public health

That the city might be the most suitable base upon which to build a public health movement is not a new idea. In the nineteenth century in Europe and North America, the rapid growth of industrial towns created the conditions under which epidemic disease was rife and it was the cities that responded to the challenge. During that era it was common for public health initiatives at the city level to be local government responsibilities. The development of large bureaucracies based on the administration of medical care services came later.

Today the city with its own political mandate and often highly developed sense of civic pride is again uniquely placed to develop the kind of citizen-responsive health promotion initiatives which are necessary to tackle the new health problems of the twenty-first century. As the most decentralised administrative level which can marshall the necessary resources and which has wide-ranging responsibilities and networks, the city is in an ideal position to support the type of inter-sectoral process which leads to creative, effective and efficient action.

Within Europe, cities are now to be found at many different stages of development. In some parts, new cities are still being established and old ones continue to grow or to be remodelled. In other parts, once great cities are in a state of crisis and apparent rapid decline. Despite prophecies that the cities are doomed, they remain in the front line of innovation and change; they continue to be the focus for the energies of youth and for many of our dreams of an urban Utopia. The challenge is to find ways of renewing the momentum towards achieving a high quality of life and 'Health for All' for city dwellers.

The familiar trends of growth and decay in cities have occurred in parallel with changes in traditional social structures – the decline of the three generation family and the changing status of marriage, redefinition of relations between the sexes and many changes in personal and social expectations. Cities as the contexts in which so many people live out their lives have come to reflect the growing tensions and conflicting aspirations between those individuals and groups which inhabit them.

Traditional matters for concern, which include unemployment, housing, education, environmental and occupational health and disease, are still with us, but in different and more subtle forms. Each of the traditional areas of public health needs to be re-examined from a present-day perspective; quality of life and aesthetics are now as important as quantity and function. The limitations of a mechanistic view of health, which ignores these perspectives, are now becoming apparent.

A number of lessons can be learned from the old public health. The first is that the important problems are usually obvious, although often overlooked or misunderstood in ways which prevent effective remediable action. Because of the current scientific theory that cholera was caused by bad air, John Snow in London in 1854 had great difficulty in persuading the authorities to remove the handle from the contaminated Broad Street water pump. In insisting that the handle be removed, Snow demonstrated that public health must be pragmatic, opportunistic and confident, perhaps taking action before the causal links have been confirmed. Today's Broad Street pumps include: the association between heart disease and excess production and marketing of animal fat products; the association between a range of health problems in young people including alcohol and drug abuse; and the economic and social conditions of young people in Europe at the present time.

Health advocacy – to be a trouble-maker for health – came to be one of the functions of public health practitioners in some parts of Europe in the last century; that function needs to be revived or rediscovered today.

Similarly, the important lesson that, in public health, communication must reach the whole population, means that populist use of media and forms of publication are essential; this includes information on the health of the population itself so that the community may play an informed part in setting its own priorities and holding its public services to account.

Outline of the project. The Healthy City Project is intended to last for 5 years by which time the aim will be that practical models of health promotion at the city level will be commonplace in the thirty-three European countries that are member states of

WHO. The role of WHO is to act as a catalyst in the process of setting a new health agenda, raising public awareness of the new public health issues and establishing models of good practice. By providing technical support to a small number of collaborating cities and creating opportunities for these cities to share their experiences it is planned to pilot approaches which will have a widespread applicability (Ashton *et al.* 1986; Barnard 1986; Ashton 1986b).

Since the project began in 1986, WHO has been working with up to twenty-one cities in workshops and through technical support at the officer level to assist cities in developing broad-based city health plans. Because of the overwhelming level of interest in the project, a second phase in which national networks of collaborating cities are established, began to occur even during the first year. The collaborating cities will play an important part in furthering the development of these networks through the organisation of national conferences and workshops. The centrepiece of the project from the point of view of information exchange between cities is to be an annual International Healthy Cities Symposium which will provide an opportunity for large numbers of cities to share in the experiences of others and become involved in the project themselves.

The project is backed up by WHO supporting centres in Liverpool and Gothenberg which are responsible for generating a range of materials of assistance to participating cities and facilitating research and teaching related to the project. The materials will include background papers, a resource pack, details of city health plans and model programmes, books, newsletters and reports.

A central output will be a European collaborative television series on the Healthy City. The information and data provided by participating cities will be the basis for collation and comparison of indicators, strategies and true stories. It is through all of these activities that WHO hope to give a major thrust towards the realisation of the new public health.

Steps towards a healthy city

The Healthy Cities Project contains five major elements:
    1. The formulation of concepts leading to the adoption of city health plans which are action-based.
    2.The development of models of good practice. These will represent a variety of different entry points into action to achieve a Healthy City depending on the cities own health

priorities. These may range from major environmental action to programmes designed to support individual change in life-styles and will illustrate the principles of Health Promotion.

3. Monitoring and research into the effectiveness of models of good practice on health in cities.

4. Dissemination of ideas and experiences between collaborating cities and other interested cities.

5. Mutual support, collaboration and learning between the cities of Europe.

Based on experience so far, and on lessons to be drawn from the old public health, the following initiatives are being encouraged as part of the project:

(i) The production of a corporate health plan for the city which is based on a community diagnosis and represents collaboration between the relevant governmental and non-governmental bodies within the city. This plan should incorporate a commitment to participation and multi-sectoral approach and to the indentification of city health goals based on action strategies in line with WHO philosophy.

(ii) The establishment of an inter-sectoral Healthy Cities Committee as a decision-making committee of the city council.

(iii) The establishment of an interdepartmental officer group to implement the health plan and to advise on the health aspects of city policies through the production of Health Impact Statements.

(iv) Exploring ways in which the Health Advocacy function can be established within the city.

(v) The generation of a broad-based public debate about the creation of a Healthy City.

These initiatives need to be informed by appropriate data on the health of the city and it is expected that a new health data base will be created based on the indicators identified as useful by the WHO collaborating cities. These will need to be complemented by population health surveys of at least the most disadvantaged groups of the population to assess their well-being and obtain the true stories of their health risks, e.g. the unemployed, women, immigrants and ethnic minorities. Appropriate support should be sought from local academic institutions in addressing the research questions which emerge from planning for health in the city.

The emphasis of these initiatives is on the provision of enabling mechanisms for health promotion to be developed through healthy public policy and increased public accountability. They should demonstrate a commitment to public participation in health issues and a willingness to address the issues of equity in health. It is expected that cities will wish to develop close working relationships with the local media to inform the public about the city's state of health and the initiatives which might be taken to improve it.

It seems likely that a wide variety of ideas and lessons will be generated by this project particularly in relation to public participation and inter-sectoral co-operation. There is clearly a great deal of scope at the city level for developing health promotion policies and activity in all the departments and institutions which are under the control of local government and for using such institutions as museums, art galleries, schools and colleges as vehicles for mass public education and involvement; a city's own public health history is itself often a powerful focus for debate and learning.

Getting started. Experience so far has suggested that firm political commitment to developing a corporate plan for city health is an essential for getting started. However, it is not uncommon to find a history of poor communication between the different sectors which need to work together, either because of political differences or because of personality or professional conflicts. The Healthy City Project itself seems to provide a kind of neutral gameboard suitable for bringing together those agencies which should share a common interest in the health of the city.

A three-step approach to getting started has much to commend it:

Step 1. A presentation from a member of the Healthy City Planning Group or from a representative from a city already involved in the project.

Step 2. The initial presentation leads to the setting up of a small interdepartmental working group to explore the feasibility of a healthy cities project and identify the problems; commonly the environmental health and city planning departments are involved at this stage.

Step 3. The establishment of a health policy sub-committee with a brief to take forward the healthy cities project and to establish a broad-based officer group to produce a community diagnosis and begin the process of drafting a discussion document which will form the basis of a corporate health plan for the city.

References

Ashton, J. (1986) *A healthy Liverpool (vision or dream)*, (background paper for the Healthy Cities Symposium, Lisbon, Portugal), Copenhagen: WHO.

Ashton, J., Grey, F. and Barnard, K. (1986a) Healthy cities – WHO's new public health initiative, *Health Promotion 1*, 319–24.

Ashton, J., Seymour, H., Ingledew, D., Ireland, R., Hopley, E., Parry, A., Ryan, M., and Holbourn, A. (1986a) Promoting the new public health in Mersey, *Health Education Journal 45*, 174–9.

Barnard, K. (1986) Lisbon Healthy Cities Symposium, Notes of closing address on behalf of the planning group. Copenhagen: WHO.

Hancock, T. and Duhl, L. J. (1986) Healthy cities; promoting health in the urban context, (A background working paper for the Healthy Cities Symposium, Lisbon, Portugal, Copenhagen: WHO.

Kickbusch, I. (1986) Health Promotion; A Global Perspective, key-note address, Canadian Public Health Association 77th Annual Conference, Health Promotion Strategies for Action, *Canadian Journal of Public Health 77*, 321–6.

Lalonde, M. (1974) *A New Perspective on the Health of Canadians*, Canada: Minister of Supply and Services.

McKeown, T. (1976) *The Role of Medicine, Dream, Mirage or Nemesis?*, Nuffield Provincial Hospitals Trust.

Vertio H. (1986). Healthy Cities. Promoting Health in the Urban Context. Dimensions and indicators. A background working paper for the 'Healthy Cities Symposium' Lisbon, Portugal, (1986). W.H.O Copenhagen.

World Health Organisation (1981) *Global Strategy for Health For All By the Year 2000*, Geneva: WHO.

World Health Organisation (1984) *Health Promotion*, A discussion document on the concept and principles, Copenhagen: WHO.

World Health Organisation (1981) *Regional Strategy for Attaining Health For All by the Year 2000*, EUr/RC 30 8 Rev. 1, Copenhagen: WHO.

World Health Organisation (1986) *Targets for Health For All 2000*, Copenhagen: WHO.

World Health Organisaton/Health and Welfare, Canada/Canadian Public Health Association (1986) *Ottawa Charter for Health Promotion*.

25

PAULINE GINNETY, JANE WILDE AND MARY BLACK

PARTICIPATION IN PRACTICE: AN EXAMPLE FROM BELFAST

Introduction

Since the Declaration of Alma Ata in 1978 (WHO) the 'Health for All' (HFA) philosophy has received fairly widespread acceptance. For it to become a reality there is a clear need for multi-sectoral co-operation: healthy public policies; changes in work practices and in the training of health and social workers – *all* of which should be underpinned by a firm belief in the concept of lay participation.

The importance of lay participation in achieving the HFA goals cannot be underestimated, and attention needs to be given to methods of fostering it. Over the past few years, experience has been building up on how to turn the philosophy into practice and it seems timely, therefore, to start sharing experiences. While doing this we should also be talking about those things which hindered, as well as helped, the process.

Lay participation is dependent on professional recognition of lay competence in health, and will require health workers to overcome the effects of their professional training to acknowledge this. Therefore, in addition to changing professional training approaches, it is essential that mechanisms are developed which help health workers and lay people to identify barriers to participation and find ways of overcoming them at a local level.

This paper describes a practical example which encouraged lay participation in health by the development of a Health Profile (Ginnety *et al.*, 1985) in a small neighbourhood called Moyard.

The approach was community-based with health and social workers acting as facilitators.

The Profile was used to: bring lay people and professionals together on an equal footing, relying as it did on the experience of both groups; identify local health issues and propose changes which could improve health or the conditions affecting health locally; provide information for both the community and professionals; and to encourage policymakers to understand and recognise the implications of 'Health For All'.

The outcome has been used not only to press for lay participation in the planning process of local health services but also to try to influence planning in other sectors such as the Northern Ireland Housing Executive and the Department of the Environment, which are central agencies undertaking many of the functions of local government.

The development of the Moyard Health Profile

Moyard is a small, multiply-deprived housing estate in West Belfast. The profile was initiated as a response by the Eastern Health and Social Services Board (EHSSB) to a request from the Moyard Housing Action Group. They were campaigning for the demolition of flats in the estate and were very concerned about a range of health problems associated with the environment, such as outbreaks of gastroenteritis, which were affecting children in Moyard. They had previously lobbied other public service agencies without success.

The Board asked our small group (which comprised a health visitor, community worker, social worker, community physician and health education officer) to work with members of the Moyard community to establish a health profile of the estate. We had recently formed as a group, and had just started exploring ways of identifying health needs in small areas. Apart from a common belief in lay participation and a commitment to health promotion, we had not refined our ideas and did not feel very well equipped for the task. However, we recognised that this opportunity represented a significant chance to translate the rhetoric of lay participation into practice so we took it. The result was the formation of a group comprising community members and ourselves who eventually carried out a door-to-door health survey of the estate, according to the wishes of the community, and we subsequently compiled a report.

The survey and its results will not be discussed, because the *process* is more relevant here. Suffice it to say that the report was widely distributed and used to press for changes in service provision in the area. It also became a local focus for discussion about the concepts of multisectoral co-operation and lay participation in health.

Factors which influenced the process. With the benefits of hindsight we recognise a number of factors which assisted the process and also some pitfalls which may have been unavoidable at the time but which should be anticipated by anyone who intends to work in this particular way.

One of the first things needed was to gain wide community support for any initiative that would be taken in the area and, for that, a representative group was essential. As anyone who has ever attempted to form a representative group knows, it is not a simple process. However, we were fortunate in two respects: (1) the existence of a well organised Housing Action Group on the estate; and (2) the group had a very experienced community worker as a member. The community worker followed up contacts identified by the Housing Action Group as well as meeting recognised community leaders. She also arranged to meet other people whose names cropped up in conversation and who were deeply involved in the community. A public meeting was arranged to introduce us to the community in order to outline the task and look for community support. The groundwork which was done in preparation for this meeting was crucial to the formation of a truly representative group. As a result, a wide range of people who did not otherwise have a high public profile attended the meeting, as well as recognised local leaders. Several people who were at the meeting volunteered to join what became known as The Moyard Health Profile Group. This group developed a plan of action: they designed and administered a questionnaire to all households on the estate; they produced a report and communicated its findings to the Moyard community and to the Eastern Health and Social Services Board.

The success of this process was demonstrated by the willing co-operation of the community in the gathering of information and their satisfaction with the outcome. When the report emerged at the end of two turbulent years, all the original members plus a few additional people were active in the group and were keen to continue on into the next stage.

We recognised that the location and timing of meetings must be suitable for local people, so the group met on a regular basis at a set day and time in the open area of the youth club on the estate. Local people felt comfortable about coming into the youth club and joining the meetings, which were informal and friendly. (If health premises had been sited on the estate we might have chosen to meet there: however, this would probably have been a mistake, as we found that the local people perceived health premises as unfriendly.)

It is important to agree to a shared agenda for action at the outset, thus ensuring that everyone is pursuing the same goal. In this case the agreement was to undertake a household survey on the estate.

We found that, although the professionals in the group were committed to lay participation, some had difficulty in restraining themselves from rushing ahead and taking over. Fortunately, the lay members were suitably assertive when this happened. For example, in the development of the questionnaire, two members volunteered to draft it and then presented it to the group as a *fait accompli*. It was rejected by the lay members and was subsequently redesigned by the whole group working together. This formed a useful learning point.

Lessons learnt. The biggest difficulty we experienced was in our relationship with local Health and Social Services (H&SS) management and workers. Although the Health Profile had been commissioned by the Board, it was viewed with some suspicion by local management and, as a result, local field-workers from health and social services were unable to be involved. This resulted in difficulties in gaining access to child health records, lack of clerical support and accommodation.

In summary, the lessons learnt from this experience were:

(i) There is need for sensitive and thorough groundwork at a number of levels particularly with: the local community; the local management to gain commitment; and local health and social workers to gain co-operation.

(ii) A clearly defined agreed agenda is essential.

(iii) Facilities in which members of the community feel 'comfortable' should be used for meetings.

(iv) The professionals who are involved should have a firm knowledge and commitment to lay participation.

The development of lay participation in planning

The Moyard Report was published in May 1985. It highlighted the socio-economic and environmental influences on health as perceived by the people of Moyard as well as the health experiences of the community. In addition, it emphasised the need for multisectoral co-operation at both policy-making and local levels and stressed the need for community participation in the planning and implementation of local services.

The Report generated interest and discussion with a range of groups. For example:

the Moyard community itself;
other community groups, local H&SS management and field-workers;
the EHSSB (both officers and members);
DHSS (Permanent Secretary and Minister for Health);
Belfast Co-ordinating Committee;
Northern Ireland Housing Executive;
Department of the Environment.

Within Moyard. The report was welcomed and used in many ways. For example, local groups such as the Housing Action Group felt it gave them credibility when dealing with agencies such as the Housing Executive and the Department of the Environment. On an individual basis, local people felt empowered by having access to the report and have experienced more constructive responses in their dialogue with individual agencies since it was published.

Other public agencies. The Health Profile Group held a meeting with representatives from the other sectors and used the Report to encourage discussion. Many of the representatives did not know each other and some had never been on the estate before. They displayed little enthusiasm for working together let alone encouraging lay participation. Unfortunately, nothing lasting, by way of multisectoral co-operation, came out of this meeting.

Local Health and Social Services (H&SS) management. Members of the Unit of Management Group met with the Health Profile Group to discuss the Report and subsequently put it on the agenda of their formal meeting. As a result, a small *ad hoc* working group was established composed of H&SS workers and members of the Moyard community, with a remit to respond appropriately to the Report.

This part of the process was important in terms of the professionals learning to consult local people about decisions to be taken regarding the Report. Incidentally, the professionals (all middle-management or field-workers) were initially resistant to lay membership of the group.

The working group reviewed progress since the Report and addressed the major recommendations. After considerable discussion it was acknowledged that Health and Social Services arrangements for the area were inadequate (for example, there were no GPs based in the local health centre) and the working group recommended the formation of a permanent Health Committee for the greater Whiterock area (of which Moyard is a part) which would be composed of local people and statutory workers.

The working group recommended that the terms of reference of the Health Committee should be to:

Participation in practice – an example from Belfast 294

1. Use Whiterock Health Centre as a focus for change by encouraging full use of its facilities and improving services to the local community;
2. Act as a bridge between residents and workers to increase mutual understanding of the health needs and services in the area;
3. Establish links with other bodies, such as the Housing Executive, the Department of Environment, Environmental Health Officers, with the aim of developing multisectoral co-operation at a local level.

In addition, the Health Committee would be expected to establish a local health information base which would be easily accessible to the community. It was envisaged that access to health data would provide a useful starting point for the community as a whole to participate in decisions about services for their community.

Because the lay members of the sub-group were selected from the Health Profile Group they were familiar with the HFA philosophy and the issue of lay participation in health as well as with the findings of the Health Profile. Some of the professionals lagged behind the lay members in these respects and this created some tension in the group.

The lay members of the group felt at a disadvantage because the meetings took place in health services' premises; this was heightened by the fact that some of the professionals felt uncomfortable about sitting down with lay people to discuss what they perceived to be internal matters.

When the Report went to the Ulster Medical Group (UMG) there was some resistance to the recommendation to set up a Health Committee. It was referred back to the EHSSB which supported the recommendation but the first meeting of the Committee has not yet been called – perhaps because of perceptions of loss of control by the UMG, duplication of work for Health and Social Services and lack of 'clear lines' of management for Health and Social Services.

Lessons learnt

(i) The acceptance of the profile at a high level (i.e. Board, DHSS) was a useful lever for local action at the beginning but this influence eventually diminished, therefore a long term strategy is needed to maintain momentum.

(ii) Work needs to be done with both management and fieldworkers – on the Community Development approach to health and on attitudes to lay participation – before a committee is formed with lay people.

(iii) Lay members need to be supported through the early stages of the group life of the Committee until they feel comfortable working with professionals. A bridge person such as a Community Development health worker is very valuable.

(iv) The Chairperson also needs support from the committee to cope with bringing the two groups together and achieving an outcome.

(v) Committed individuals are needed to carry on the work in the community so it is essential that local workers are involved.

(vi) Representatives from other sectors need to be involved in discussion about the HFA philosophy and lay participation before becoming involved in projects with local people, particularly if they do not perceive health as an obvious part of their role or function.

Possibilities for the future

As well as continuing to support the formation and activity of this Health Committee it is important to move towards assisting in the establishment of other health profiles. We now feel that the pre-requisites for starting a health profile are:

(a) community demand, i.e. the existence of individuals or groups concerned about health in their community;

(b) readiness of local workers in the health, social and community work-field to become involved;

(c) support from management (HSS) and commitment to lay participation in health;

(d) training opportunities for staff;

(e) supportive policy;

(f) multidisciplinary/multisectoral co-operation.

Overall, most of these requirements can be met and initial discussions are currently under way for another health profile to be commenced. The community in question has already been involved in health initiatives and there is a core of lay people with an interest in health. Local health workers have been involved in a facilitative way in these initiatives and are committed to developing the concept of lay participation in health. Health and Social Services management is sympathetic and one member of the UMG has offered practical assistance which it is felt will be supported by her management colleagues. With regard to policies, both the Regional Strategic Plan (DHSS, 1987) and the Area Operational Plan (EHSSB, 1987) show clear commitment to the 'Health for All' philosophy. In addition, the Board and other public sector agencies made strong representations to the WHO to have Belfast included in the 'Healthy Cities' project. Belfast has now been invited to participate in the 'Healthy Cities' project. Their commitment to this project should make it easier for workers from all sectors to work together at a local level. It is felt that ward-based Health Profiles would be valuable in providing local networks and information for the subject.

Conclusion

The lessons learnt and outlined in this paper will form part of a plan for the next profile and assist in achieving the aim of reorienting the health service, developing multisectoral co-operation and ensuring lay participation in the planning and implementation of health services.

The overriding lesson for us in developing the Moyard Health Profile was that the process takes a long time and results are not seen overnight. As Donnison (1987) says about the community based approach: 'it has been developed – sometimes as an act of desperation – in order to solve problems which defeated conventional services operating in conventional ways'. We feel that the Moyard Health Profile was born out of an attempt to solve problems which had defeated conventional approaches and has served to demonstrate that lay participation is an important step which must be taken if community health issues are to be addressed in an appropriate way. The process is slow and arduous and requires tenacity on the part of those involved to overcome barriers, ranging from hostility to bureaucratic inertia, both of which can bring the process to a standstill. Most of all it needs committed lay people who can endure the soul-searching in which professionals engage over what must appear to be the essentially simple issue of the rights of lay people to be involved in decisions which affect their health.

References

The Alma Ata Conference on Primary Health Care, *WHO Chronicle* 1978, 409–30
DHSS Regional Strategic Plan (NI) 1987.
Donnison D., The Community Based Approach, 1987.
EHSSB Area Operational Plan 1987.
Ginnety, P., Black, M. and Kelly, K., The Moyard Health Profile, EHSSB 1985.

26

CHRISTEL ZENKER AND ROSEMARIE KLESSE

HEALTH MEETING CENTRES IN BREMEN

The Bremen Institute for Prevention Research and Social Medicine
(BIPS) is one of five study centres of the multicentre German
Cardiovascular Prevention Study (GCP), which is funded by
the Federal Ministry of Research and Technology until 1991.
This paper describes the background to, and work of, two health-
meeting centres in Bremen.

Aims of the meeting centres

The German Cardiovascular Prevention Study encompasses two
rather different approaches. On the one hand, the aim of the study
is to reduce cardiovascular disease (mainly myocardial infarction
and stroke) within the 20–69 age group by reducing relevant
risk factors in the population. Health education and standardised risk-factor programmes are regarded as the most appropriate
methods for this, as individual behavioural change is the desired
outcome. For example, it is hoped that by 1991 as many citizens
as possible will have changed their behavioural patterns, will prefer
a healthier diet, will have normal blood pressure, not be overweight, smoke less and engage in a lot of physical exercise. On
the other hand, the prevention programme is based on community-
oriented health promotion; the aim being to strengthen healthy
lifestyles in the whole community. This includes supporting self-
responsibility and self-help activities in the community by as many
structural changes as possible. The aim, then, is that the citizens of
Bremen should, with the help of experts, develop a new consciousness about health and create a 'healthy city' of their own; instead

297

of being passive health consumers, the citizens should favour active participation in health promotion.

The main intervention aims in Bremen are marked by:

1. *Direct co-operation with citizens and self-help groups:* this refers principally to individual strategies for solving problems.

2. *A close co-operation with other community-based institutions:* this includes traditional health organisations such as medical associations, hospitals, health offices, counselling boards and compulsory sickness funds. Other important institutions within the community with whom co-operation is sought include schools, adult education centres, companies, political institutions and churches.

3. *Co-operation with 'multipliers':* this term refers to people trained to direct standardised programmes for the reduction of risk factors, physicians, and pharmacists, but also refers to restaurant owners who could be very important in bringing about certain kinds of structural changes.

4. *Co-operation with the mass media:* this is necessary in order to facilitate the intervention work and has increased recognition of the Institute, the meeting centres and the GCP study in general.

As the Institute is located in the city centre and both the meeting centres are in the two intervention districts, Bremen-North and Bremen-West, the two sets of staff have rather different fields of activity.

The Bremen Institute for Prevention Research and Social Medicine (BIPS)

The staff of the Institute are, above all, responsible for the co-ordination of the intervention work within the intervention areas and also for activities, in general, in the Bremen area. These activities include the co-ordination and implementation of programmes and courses relating to risk factors, the training of 'multipliers' and the design of interventions such as programmes for healthier eating. Another essential part of the Institute's work is the production of information packs on topics such as risk factors or salt content of canned foods. A general health guide which gives information about all the health programmes offered in Bremen has also been compiled. The staff of the Institute have also initiated a health 'task force', which comprises the most important representatives of all health institutions in the city. Co-operation with the mass media is co-ordinated by the Institute which also has responsibility for the evaluation of the intervention programme.

The meeting centres

The main intervention activities of the meeting centres include:

    Counselling of citizens
    Monitoring of health initiatives in the community
    Co-operation with the local institutions
    Participation in community life
    Co-operation with the local mass media
    Documentation of the Centres' work regarding contact within the community.

When the two centres began their work it was necessary to find out, first, what the citizens' health needs were and, second, what the working aims of institutions within the community were. In order to be integrated in the community, it was also essential to find co-operating partners for this work so that the meeting centres would serve as a platform for all health needs.

Within our work concept, we regard cardiovascular health as being part of general social, physical and psychic health. Thus, each risk factor of any individual is an expression of his or her individual lifestyle. Understanding these lifestyles and finding possibilities for changing them is seen as one key to better health in the community. In this way, our work can be seen as part of a general process of health promotion.

Location and design of the meeting centres. We rented shops with large windows situated on busy streets in the centres of Bremen-North and Bremen-West. In order to encourage people to come in we tried to design the rooms and windows in a casual way. We try to keep the Centres free from our personal or political opinions and have produced a folder containing a photograph of the staff, and which describes the most important fields of our work. There are four staff members; not all work full time.

The work of the meeting centres. In 1986 we made almost 5,700 counselling contacts with citizens and almost 700 contacts with institutions and organisations. The main topics of the counselling already provided by the centres refer to risk factors, but often reveal social, emotional or economic problems. In discussing these problems with the visitors, we try to throw some light on the background to the risk factors and assist them in working out a solution that is acceptable to them (help for self-help) such as: joining a self-help group; joining a group offering a standardised programme; or seeking specific counselling.

The contacts with institutions and organisations have different purposes. These are primarily to get to know each other by exchanging information about the nature and aims of our respective activities, in order to reduce possible fears about the Centres as a new institution in the community (and vice versa) and, secondly, to find co-operation partners. We have found that while it is easy to do work with counselling boards, institutions of adult education, churches and local government offices, it is difficult to do work in companies, factories and schools. Some of the reasons for this are structural problems such as hierarchy, lack of competence, and competition between institutions within companies. Our most difficult experience, however, was trying to co-operate with physicians and hospital doctors.

From the beginning, we took part in community activities such as local festivals so that we could reach the people who do not come to the Centres. These are mainly foreigners, unemployed young people and those of lower social class. We believe that since they do not come to the Centres, we must go to the places where they live and meet them.

Co-operation with the local newspapers is very good. For example, they publish articles on a regular basis and announcements for us as often as desired, completely free of charge.

The rest of our work is conducted in other ways and includes:

    Cooking with unemployed young people

    Health festivals in 'social problem' areas

    Relaxation classes with Turkish women

    Offering counselling sessions in the Town Hall.

The different fields of our many activities represent the general ideas of our work and from this we derived our slogan 'Healthier living – a matter of the heart'.

Problems of community-based health promotion

Initiating health promotion within the community can be problematic and may lead to a number of difficulties. First, the work is very time-consuming and the work-load is not constant. Therefore, it has to be designed according to the continuously changing needs within the comunity. The experience of the staff has to be constantly adapted to changing conditions in the working process. Second, there are few transferable experiences from other studies and, third, it is proving difficult to reach all social classes. Our work in the Centres will ultimately be judged in terms of the overall aim of the study – namely, a reduction in cardiovascular mortality. Therefore, possible selection regarding social class participation must be considered. A final difficulty relates to the incorporation, once the study is completed, of the Centres into the community – structurally and conceptually.

Three possible future directions are being considered:

(i) the taking over of the Centres by the community, although this would not be easy either financially or politically; or

(ii) the taking over of the Centres by non-profit associations such as welfare organisations; or

(iii) starting a new project in 1989 to evaluate the community-oriented health promotion already begun by the health meeting centres.

It remains to be seen if the aims of the meeting centres, namely a self-responsible understanding of health, can be achieved within the short time available for the study. At present, understanding of health is still characterised in terms of illness prevention through experts rather than by health consciousness on the part of the citizens.

27

DAVID CILL-MHUIRE

THE COMMUNITY HEALTH RESOURCE UNIT:
A LOCAL INITIATIVE IN GLASGOW

The Community Health Resource Unit is based in an area in the North East of Glasgow. Local people call this area 'Royston' although a more accurate title might be 'The Royston Corridor' since this is the local authority planners' official designation for the area. Local people, however, don't usually go along with this official designation, preferring to stick to their historically grounded and organic understanding of the various communities which together make up the planners' statistically constructed supra-community which is the 'Royston Corridor'. The 'Corridor', in fact, comprises three major communities – namely Roystonhill, Germiston and Blackhill.

The area has traditionally been a poor one, characterised by high unemployment and other statistical indicators of deprivation including bad public health. Indeed it is interesting to remember that Blackhill was originally built as a tuberculosis colony. To this day the 'Corridor' continues to manifest high indices of socio-economic deprivation; it continues to suffer from a lack of social resources and economic investment; and this material deprivation is reflected in the area's appalling public/community health record.

Why the unit was established

Strathclyde Regional Council, which administers services for a large part of the west of Scotland, had been aware for some years of the discrepancies in the socio-economic and health-performance indices in multiply deprived areas, compared to the more residential and professional parts of the city of Glasgow. It established

302

both its concern, and its desire, to tackle these socially generated health inequalities in its policy document – 'Social Strategy
for the Eighties'. As well as continuing to co-operate with the
various Health Boards in its constituency via the Joint Liaison
Committees, Strathclyde Regional Council also actively sought to
pilot some kind of alternative public or community-based health
intervention that would be complementary to the medical model
of the National Health Service as expressed through the medium
of the various Health Boards. The Region's Community Development Committee, therefore, commissioned the Community Projects Foundation to produce a consultative report on the potential
for a community development approach to health promotion in the
depressed areas within its boundaries and in Glasgow in particular.
This report confirmed the potential of such an approach in tackling
socially-generated health issues in the deprived areas and, given
that the 'Corridor' is representative of these areas' experiences, the
Unit was sited in the Social Work Area Office in Royston.

The Region was concerned that the limited impact of health
promotion interventions, in areas such as Royston, was due to
the tendency of such programmes towards individualising their
message when attempting to alter behaviour patterns amongst the
people while taking little or no notice of the concrete conditions,
needs, and priorities of the populace residing in these communities.
In short, and without wishing to decry the phenomenal gains in general health standards made by the NHS and other health promotion
agencies, the Region and the Community Projects Foundation were
concerned that health had been abstracted from its social context
by some health professionals, and that these practitioners were,
therefore, to some degree, out of touch with the concrete realities
of health care and promotion. In other words, many practitioners
seemed to be ignoring the fact that there is a material social basis
for the state of the individual's health, and that the professionals,
therefore, failed to recognise that this individual experience is a
manifestation of the collective human condition within the impoverished working-class housing schemes.

The Unit's funders were unhappy that the public dimension
to health improvement and maintenance seemed to have been
largely abandoned in favour of a more limited individualistic,
clinical perspective and, as such, there had been a retreat from
the creative, visionary and holistic endeavours of the early public
health pioneers.

The Unit was, therefore, conceived and designed by Strathclyde
Regional Council and the Community Projects Foundation, as the

antithesis to the dominant pathological, individualistic, 'cultural imperialist' or the 'we're telling you' style of health promotion that seems to be endemic in some health service and local authority practice in deprived communities.

There is an old Chinese proverb which neatly sums up the Unit's view of the current state of the art in front-line health promotion, and this roughly translates as follows: 'It is better to walk with two legs than one.' Or to put it in other words, we need a public model of health as well as the currently favoured medical model. We need a collective or social point of reference as a context for the diagnosis of the individual's health dysfunction; and we need the lay-person's involvement as well as the professionals', if the health of the populace is to continue to improve across the various social classes, and within deprived communities in particular.

The importance of local perceptions

The people of Royston would define the area in a different way from the planners and the policy makers. This is an important point in the context of community development. The difference between the language and vision of the professionals and the ordinary person living in areas like the 'Royston Corridor', has a bearing on the efficacy of official interventions – be they housing initiatives, health promotion programmes, social work or community development interventions. If such programmes are to be effective, then practitioners need to be aware of the view of local people, and they need to incorporate them into their interventions. Thus, initiatives need to defer to some degree to local nuances and sensibilities. This is especially true for projects like the Unit which seeks to promote public health in deprived working-class areas, where health is traditionally perceived (because of the way the various agencies have tended to promote health issues) as being something that only the better-off can afford.

If the Unit failed to take account of local perceptions, then, like so many other health promotion interventions, it would be viewed as yet another exercise in 'cultural imperialism'. Or, to put it in plain language, people would dismiss it as nonsense. It would be seen as irrelevant, because it was pedalling values and priorities that were of no relation to the everyday realities that local people have to cope with in the depressed, predominantly working-class housing schemes.

It is clear to the Unit that any meaningful community development programme or health-education/promotion intervention in areas like the 'Corridor', needs to move at the pace of the local people, and needs to be attuned to local consciousness if it is to have a real impact.

This close identification with ordinary people is central to the community development practice of the Unit, and this work model is underwritten and supported by its two major co-funders – Strathclyde Regional Council and the Community Projects Foundation. This identification also animates the Unit's approach within its other operational contexts: namely, informing local people on the policy and work practice of the local authorities, and other agencies, such as the Health Board. Indeed, this identification with ordinary people's health needs was one of the major factors behind the Unit's establishment by its funders in 1985, who were opposed to the continued imposition of foreign or alien values and priorities on the populace of the depressed schemes by outside experts, who take little or no account, of the concrete social conditions in which their patients/consumers have to live. This underpins the aims and objectives, the programmes and the community development practice, of the Unit's field-staff when working with local people, and when transmitting any lessons learned from working with local people to the appropriate policy makers and practitioners.

The work of the Community Health Resource Unit (CHRU)

The Community Health Resource Unit has a three-pronged remit:

(1) The Unit is charged with developing models of community development practice in the public/community health arena at a local level;

(2) It is remitted to tackle health issues at the level of strategic policy-making;

(3) Finally, it is required to inform and illuminate current local authority work practice by means of training programmes, and information dissemination.

However, the Unit's staffing complement is small, and consequently there is only so much we can humanly hope to achieve given the heavy demands that are generated because of our various operational commitments. In fact, the Unit comprises one senior community health worker, two basic grade community health workers, and one part-time administrator. It is therefore clear that, because of these staffing constrictions and the range of our operational tasks, we cannot address all the issues that come our way.

Nevertheless, we do attempt to demonstrate a potential and complementary model of working with health issues, both to local people and professionals, as well as to the policy makers, social planners and practitioners from a number of different disciplines in the Glasgow area. We seek to promote a social or public model of health amongst the relevant agencies, and we attempt to encourage joint work on an equal basis between them: we facilitate these outcomes by means of our practical examples of what can be achieved, and by offering an information resource as a back-up to any interested parties on a Glasgow-wide basis, as well as at a local Royston level.

The remainder of this paper considers some practical examples of the three tiers of the Unit's operations:

Local field-work. As discussed previously, it is necessary to avoid the 'we'll tell you what the score is' approach, which if pursued, would result in a loss of credibility, with local people dismissing it as being of no value to them. Field-work is a crucial context in which to avoid this kind of method of working with people.

Thus, the key to effective community development work on a local level is, in the first place, drawing out of people their perceptions about local health needs and priorities and in the second place, winning their confidence in the process. Subsequently, they can be helped to identify the broader issues which they may not have considered previously, or which they were only dimly aware of because of other demands on their time and energies.

Community development field-work, therefore, attempts to bring people together around issues of common interest, and it tries to help them determine the course of action they may wish to take. It is for them – because they have to endure the conditions – to decide on the methods for resolving the situation and, if community development is to be both effective and legitimate in their eyes, then it must take cognisance of this truth.

There are a number of examples which would serve to illuminate this style of work. For example: work with the local tenants organisations, work with women and tranquillisers, work with campaigning groups against hospital closures, etc. In this instance I will briefly use the local Community Health Plan Group (CHPG) as an example, because it illustrates how local people come together to tell the professionals (for a change) what the needs and priorities of the area are.

Although the CHPG is still a relatively new local group (composed of delegates from the Pensioners Action Group, the Northern Disabled Action Group, Rosemount Mothers and Toddlers Group, and the Local Health Council amongst others) it has already identified a range of health issues in the part of the

'Corridor' it covers. These amount to several pages worth of concerns. The members are now beginning to prioritise, investigate and articulate these issues in a more orderly fashion. They will then collate and produce the issues in the form of a local Community Health Plan which the members will use when tackling the Health Board and the relevant local authority.

Issues have been identified in a number of ways, and a range of techniques will be utilised when investigating them further. In identifying local concerns, members have exchanged and noted their own experiences, have passed on to the group the views of their colleagues in the organisations which they represent, and will be utilising surveys, for example, to identify other needs in their locality. The role of the professional in this group is now subordinate and supportive, because this is how the locally composed membership wants it.

Thus the Unit, originally having been the catalyst which led this group to become established, has now the lower profile of resourcing it on a regular basis. Other professionals assist the group on a needs basis. The members of this group come from a number of organisations in the locality, and while they are happy to draw on the practical support of various professionals in the area, they are clear that it is the views of local people that are primary in this exercise. This is the kind of independent thinking that the Unit is designed to encourage, although it has to be said that, in this instance, the membership had already come to this conclusion of their own volition.

Strategic. There are again a number of examples of the Unit's work in this arena, but in choosing to describe our work with the shop stewards, at British Rail Maintenance Limited, in producing a Health and Social Audit of the redundant work-force, a number of other facets of strategic importance can be touched on. This piece of work illustrates a kind of community development intervention that tends to be an exception to the rule in that rather than only concentrating on a geographical community, it also reaches out across physical boundaries and works with a community of interests.

In this case, the interests are the costs of such a large-scale closure to: the local and macro economy; the local state and government departments like the DHSS; the Health Service; and, of course, the consequences for the individuals themselves who have been affected in a number of ways, including suffering from adverse long-term effects on their health. The investigation of these interests is – according to the shop stewards that we work with – 'of value to the Labour Movement, and any other (geographical) working-class community which may be faced with the same kind of devastation in the future'.

This example also illustrates a fairly wide range of inter-disciplinary collaboration since the core team consists of field-staff from the Unit, the Social Work Department, Health Education, and the Department of Community Medicine, who can draw on the expertise of 'satellite' specialists.

This particular piece of work also poses questions of a strategic nature, as far as the Health Board and the appropriate local authorities are concerned. The experiences of the team, for example, have taught us a lesson about the need to be realistically aware of what constitutes a real, as opposed to a rhetorical, commitment on the part of our respective managements to workers getting involved in a sensitive issue like this. The answer must be that where the authority countenances this kind of initiative, it may also cover its options by encouraging other departments and the staff to either boycott the initiative or to work in opposition to it behind the scenes. Thus the authority has its cake and eats it too.

It is also clear to us that the Health Boards have no strategic orientation, or commitment to involving time, staff, or major resources in any coherent way in inter-disciplinary, 'pro-active' initiatives of this kind. On the contrary, and with the exception of Health Education's invaluable contribution, the boards seem intent on standing apart in some kind of splendid apolitical isolation when this kind of major socio-economic disaster and consequent public health crisis occurs.

Indeed the deafening silence emanating from health boards affected by the British Rail Maintenance Limited redundancies was only a repeat performance of their lack of comment over other major closures in Scotland over the last few years. This is surely a curious and contradictory strategic posture for a public service that is so vociferous about its cost-effectiveness and is so keen not to see costs escalate. However, it should be clearly emphasised that the health boards are not alone in this kind of passive collusion. For example, there was no involvement from the District Council beyond the sympathetic offers of information from one or two individuals; there was no involvement from the Scottish Trades Union Council despite canvassing; and to date no major strategic policy/resources support from the Regional Council, or Greater Glasgow Health Board, for their staff. The Community Education Service even withdrew from the team in the early stages of the initiative.

One has to conclude, at this point, that despite the institutional policy rhetoric about inter-agency collaboration, had it not been for the personalities concerned, this initiative would have died long ago. Nevertheless, if the team continue to be as dogged as they have been, then this piece of joint 'pro-active' practice may yet have an effect on the current policy and practice of the agencies which the members of the group represent. Certainly, it is clearly required in areas like Royston, and is needed in initiatives like this one.

On the positive side it has to be said that, at local management level and at its equivalent level within the trade-union movement, certain victories (in terms of widening people's perceptions about the value of the style and content of this kind of intervention) have been won. The trade unions have been supportive towards this initiative – the 'litmus-paper' test of this support, in the trade-union context, being: the work-place shop stewards' demand from the team for a paper on the health effects of the redundancies, for presentation to a Parliamentary Select Committee presentation; and their enthusiasm for an in-depth health audit of the former work-force. This was a major breakthrough, given the traditional 'workerism' of the shop-floor arm of the trade-union movement.

If we can produce such a study, then we may yet begin to have a more wide-ranging and profound effect on the policies and strategic practices of the agencies mentioned.

Current professional practice within the Glasgow area. It is only really now that the Unit is moving into the area of impinging directly on the practice of the various professionals within the city. This is largely due to the local field-work focus of our brief for the first 2 years of our existence. However, this is not to say that the Unit has not made a contribution on this level to date; it has, but it has been of secondary importance to the local work. Excluding specific contact work with different individual professionals, teams of workers, and community groups and voluntary organisations, the major contribution from the Unit within the city's boundaries has been that of our information resource. This has, and does, offer back-up to any organisation with a public health interest in Glasgow and, increasingly of late, outwith Glasgow.

It is the Unit's intention to begin to put greater emphasis, over the coming years, on the city-wide dimension by, for example: gathering information about community/public health activity in Glasgow, collating it on our new data-base and disseminating it, perhaps via a regular news-sheet; organising training courses for local authority fieldwork staff; and also organising interdisciplinary conferences which will allow people to exchange their practical experiences, and which will seek to impinge on the policies of the relevant agencies.

Conclusion

The staff at the Unit are under no illusions about the limits on the potential of a community development approach to health in the poor areas, because of the wider socio-economic forces that are battering the people of those neglected and increasingly squalid communities. We recognise that these forces are infinitely more powerful than small-scale community development interventions like those of the Unit. At the same time, we are convinced that this kind of approach to public health improvement has an important contribution to make: in altering organisations' policies; in affecting the behaviour and expectations of the people and the professionals alike; and perhaps, ultimately, encouraging the people to clamour for progressive as opposed to the current reactionary social change. However, at the end of the day, the means and will to effect a lasting and enlightened solution to our contemporary social inequalities, lies with those amongst us who are presently most disadvantaged by the system. This potential for resolution does not lie with the community development worker.

28

NEIL DRUMMOND

EVALUATION OF A COMMUNITY HEALTH PROJECT: THE EXPERIENCE FROM WEST GRANTON, EDINBURGH

Background

The health project is located in the north of Edinburgh, in an area characterised as multiply-deprived, with unemployment running at around 40 per cent, and the majority of the housing owned by the local authority. The area covered by the project contains about 4,600 households, with a population of over 15,000.

The project's aims are to encourage local people to become aware of issues relating to health and well-being, and to participate in action to improve these qualities. Thus the project is essentially set up to respond to needs perceived in the community, not to assert standards of health determined by medical practice or government policy.

We have a full-time staff of three: a community development worker, a health visitor, and a researcher. We also have a part-time clerical assistant. The four of us are based in a primary school in the heart of the community. The project is funded by the Scottish Home and Health Department, on the condition that its operation be monitored and evaluated.

Project activities

The essential ingredient in the project's *modus operandi* is the self-help group. These are set up either by the health visitor or the community development worker, around issues described by local people as important. Currently. the following groups meet regularly:

Tranquiliser Support Group

Women and Food Group
Fruit and Vegetable Co-operative
Stress Centre
Elderly Forum

There are occasional 'one-off' activities, the most recent being a Women's Health and Fun Day. The final component in the project's work involves 'campaigns' that may run for weeks or months, with the aim of achieving change in, for example, local government or health-board practices, such that decisions taken at executive level respond to community-based representations. One recent campaign sought to improve the chiropody service for the elderly in the community.

Techniques of evaluation

This paper briefly describes the various ways in which I am attempting to research and evaluate the project, but mainly concentrates on some of the difficulties and constraints on the research encountered in the process. In no particular order, the evaluation has involved: a survey of the area, using local residents as interviewers, asking about health status and social and environmental factors perceived as affecting people's health; collecting various forms of routine health-board data to build into a profile of the area; interviewing people involved with the project; attempting to record the day-to-day activities; monitoring telephone calls, and recording referrals to specific groups from external agencies. In principle, these are standard techniques of evaluative research. In practice, it is a feature of the context of such a health project that substantial modifications are made in the rigor of the research, in a trade-off between the demands of research for data of minimum ambiguity, and the demands of the project workers to be allowed to operate without the restrictions created by 'observation'. It was made clear by the management committee of the project when I took up the post, that 'The project is more important than the research', and I have tried to respect that injunction.

It is important, at the outset, to establish a fair basis for an evaluation of an operation like the project. Given the size of the area it has to cover, and the presence of only two workers actively engaged in community-based work, it is unreasonable to expect any measureable change in the well-being of the whole community as a result of the project's existence. Although we have carried out a large-scale health survey, and hope to repeat it in the future, its principal uses will be to guide the project toward issues of local importance in a more formal way, rather than the largely intuitive process currently occurring, and also to provide data for a numerical profile of the area.

The principal arena for evaluation is, therefore, within that group of local people who become involved with the project, and the main technique being used is, in very simple terms, for me to interview participants to find out how they became involved, what expectations they had of participation, whether these have been satisfied, and whether the experience is rated as beneficial.

There are obvious problems with this approach, since we are dealing with self-selected participants who perhaps only become involved because they saw a reasonable chance of some benefit to themselves, and having become involved, may be reluctant to criticise an activity with which they feel some identity. Using before and after interviews goes some way to overcoming this difficulty, since ex-attenders may have been dissatisfied, but may also represent 'successes' who have no further need for involvement. There is still, however, the problem of establishing that any 'benefits' experienced by people taking part in project activities are causally related to their participation.

The absence of a 'control' group may be countered by the results of the large-scale survey, and its projected repeat. If no measurable changes occur in the health status of the sample in the survey, yet improvements are reported by those involved in the project, there is a slightly stronger case for attributing those improvements to the project, rather than to a general improvement occurring throughout the community. Such conclusions would rest, quaking, on circumstantial evidence. But it is probably the best we can achieve.

This contention is supported by an attempt we made to set up a randomised controlled intervention involving parents of children under 2 years, living in a specific neighbourhood. The intention of this study was to measure, as scientifically as possible, the effectiveness of group-work as a means of informing parents about simple childhood illness, and ways of coping with it. Unfortunately only one person selected to take part in the group turned up.

The measurement of 'outcomes' leads to another difficulty: there are three basic clients for the results of the evaluation:

(1) One is the medical/scientific audience, represented particularly by the Scottish Home and Health Department. Their interest is primarily in whether the project achieves its objectives; whether it can be labelled a 'success'.

(2) The second audience for the evaluation is represented by those involved in community development. They subscribe

to the *a priori* assumption that community development is a good thing. (It would be surprising if they did not.) They are far less concerned with degrees of success or failure. They want an analysis of the processes involved. Simply, *how* does the project operate? And at the same time, their view of useful outcomes is very different from that of the medical/scientific audience. For community development workers, research should address issues of well-being, states of self-determination, 'patient-power', rather than cost effectiveness, symtomatology, or reductions in consultation rates.

(3) The third audience, the community itself, seeks both an account of how the project works *and* an indication of whether it achieves anything beneficial.

The need to satisfy the community development concern with process, raises serious problems for the researcher. One of the most useful tools for monitoring processes is, obviously, observation. But in the context of the project, there are severe restrictions on access to many project activities, given that I am male (participation is overwhelmingly female); not afflicted by an eating problem, nor on tranquilisers (other than nicotine and alcohol). Thus there are considerable areas of the project's work that are hidden from my direct sight. Whilst I am unhappy about the restrictions, I regard them as legitimate: I would not wish to encroach on, and thereby threaten, a therapeutic structure.

There are two ways of overcoming the blocks to direct observation. One is to ask the facilitators of the groups to describe the processes as they see them. Again, this raises the problem of bias; whether real or imaginary, the possibility that somebody closely identified with the activity might not give appropriate emphasis to the problems encountered renders them less than ideal as a witness.

To overcome this, in one of the groups, I asked my colleague to keep a standard record for each session, detailing information such as attendance, objectives of the meeting, whether they were achieved, etc. My hope is that by keeping this on-going record it will build into a history of the group that, on completion, will provide an account of events that will pre-empt any critical suggestion that the facilitator has edited-out problems and mistakes.

When attempting to describe the effectiveness of a specific campaign, the researcher has a better chance of gaining access. The main difficulty is to answer criticism that could be levelled, i.e. that any change that is effected would have occurred anyway, and that the project was simply lucky enough to be active on a particular topic at the right time.

To counter this, it is possible to adopt a journalistic approach, studying the history of the campaign as it appears in notes and correspondence, interviewing the key people involved in the initial stages, and then following the narrative through the hierarchy of officialdom, searching for the moments when key decisions were taken, and attempting to interview those making the decisions for 'on-the-record' accounts of the reasons *why* decisions were made in certain directions. From the project's point of view, for example, I should be looking for statements attributing decisions to the influence of the campaign.

Role of the researcher

I want to finish by describing the role of the researcher and some of the constraints inherent to it. Some are particular to the context of this project, others are more general. The dichotomy between the interests of the clients of the evaluation has already been discussed. If one side suspects you of spending too much effort on the others' interests, the inevitable result is conflict. It is vital that the researcher is sympathetic to the cause of the enterprise under study, as seen by the people most closely involved with the action. In my case, that means my colleagues: the people whose work you are investigating have got to trust you. But at the same time, research depends upon maintaining a critical point of view, of 'doubting wisely'. It is, therefore, necessary to establish oneself as a credible witness, on one's own account. It is also important to foresee the critical points of view of other audiences, and attempt to counter them. There is a story by Séan O'Faoláin that seems to me to illustrate my attitude to research in the context of a community health project, that is, of tempering enthusiasm with a critical awareness of how others might see us.

The story is about a man walking along a street at night and being tremendously attracted by the image of a room with the lights on and the curtains drawn back. He's so enchanted by the quality of the light, by the lay-out of the room, that he talks his way inside. He's carrying a full-length mirror with him, and it's too big to fit through the door, so he props it up against the hedge in the front garden. When he gets inside, however, his experience is very different. The light is flat, stale, unimpressive, and the furnishings are dull, ordinary. He's disappointed. But he happens to wander over to the window, and there, reflected in the mirror, is an image of the interior of the room, as it appears from the outside, now seen from the inside.

'Leave it there,' he says. 'It makes it more real.'

AUTHOR INDEX

SUBJECT INDEX